Praise for *The Healing Art of Essential Oils*

"Dr. Kac Young brilliantly presents a very thorough and informative book that covers everything you could want to know about essential oils … It is a must read."

—Nancy Wright, CHHC,

"[This book] contains a wealth of information about essential oil ing, compelling writing style prompts the reader to keep turning

—Lisa Tenzin-Dolma, former ... K

"With expert knowledge [Young] blends history, alchemy, and practicality into an inviting book filled with accessible ways to enjoy and benefit from venturing back to your senses with these oils. You couldn't ask for a finer guide."

—Jeannine Wiest, author of *The Alchemy of Self Healing*

"Dr. Kac Young gives us everything we could possibly want or need to know about the value of using essential oils … It's a keeper."

—Jacklyn Zeman, actress who played Nurse Bobbie on *General Hospital*

"Kac Young has outdone herself in the extensive research, compilation, and writing of her newest book … exceptionally well done."

—Terry Cole-Whittaker, author, minister, and founder of Terry Cole-Whittaker Ministries and Adventures in Enlightenment

"I have fallen in love with this book of practical wisdom! Kac offers a masterfully written guide on how to tap into the many healing properties of essential oils."

—Terah Kathryn Collins, bestselling author of *The Western Guide to Feng Shui*

"Kac Young is a poetic and thorough guide … Her book offers major wisdom and wonderfully organized and exhaustive information on both the subtle and profound healing offered with the alchemical magic of essential oils."

—Amy Leigh Mercree, author of *Joyful Living*

"A great, comprehensive book about oils. Kac has obviously done her homework. [An] amazing piece of work!"

—Rob Spears and Brenda Michaels, hosts of Conscious Talk Radio

"Fascinating, comprehensive, and insightful, [this book] will draw you into the powerful art of healing aromatherapy."

—Atherton Drenth, author of *The Intuitive Dance*

"[Kac Young's] recipes offer fresh combinations for a multitude of health issues and her deep knowledge of the oils keeps us attached to ancient healing. This book really could change your life."

—Beth Wareham, author of *The Power of No and Hair Club Burning*

My heartfelt thanks to the entire Llewelyn Worldwide team and Angela Wix and Laura Graves for bringing this manuscript into print and distribution. They are true professionals.

About the Author

Formerly a producer and director in the television industry, Kac Young, PhD, observed the harmful effects of stress and unhealthy working conditions, leading her to earn a Doctorate in Clinical Hypnotherapy, a Doctorate in Natural Healing, and the title of Naturopathic Doctor as a third credential. She's studied health, healing, biofeedback, past-life regression, Bach flowers, and Chinese Medicine, and she's traveled to all parts of the world to study under respected healers and teachers. She runs a private practice where she consults with people who want to change their lifestyle, prolong their lives, and use as many natural products as possible in the process, helping people with weight loss, smoking cessation, and addiction therapy as well as the healing of physical conditions and chronic issues.

To Write to the Author

If you wish to contact the author or would like more information about this book, please write to the author in care of Llewellyn Worldwide, Ltd. and we will forward your request. Llewellyn Worldwide, Ltd. cannot guarantee that every letter written to the author can be answered, but all will be forwarded. Please write to:

Kac Young, PhD
℅ Llewellyn Worldwide
2143 Wooddale Drive
Woodbury, MN 55125-2989

Please enclose a self-addressed stamped envelope for reply, or $1.00 to cover costs.
If outside the USA, enclose an international postal reply coupon.

KAC YOUNG, *PhD*

THE

HEALING
ART
OF
ESSENTIAL
OILS

A GUIDE TO 50 OILS FOR
REMEDY, RITUAL, AND EVERYDAY USE

Llewellyn Publications
Woodbury, Minnesota

FIRST EDITION
First Printing, 2017

Book design by Bob Gaul
Cover design by Ellen Lawson
Cover art by iStockphoto.com/51699666/botamochi
Editing by Laura Graves
Figure on page 301 by Mary Ann Zapalac
Interior plant art by iStockphoto.com/73967279/Olgaorly
Other interior illustrations by Llewellyn art department

Llewellyn Publications is a registered trademark of Llewellyn Worldwide Ltd.

Library of Congress Cataloging-in-Publication Data
Names: Young, Kac, author.
Title: The healing art of essential oils : a guide to 50 oils for remedy, ritual, and everyday use / Kac Young, PhD.
Description: First edition. | Woodbury, Minnesota : Llewellyn Publications, [2017] | Includes bibliographical references and index.
Identifiers: LCCN 2016037295 (print) | LCCN 2016037858 (ebook) | ISBN: 9780738750477 | ISBN 9780738751733 ()
Subjects: LCSH: Essences and essential oils—Therapeutic use. | Healing. | Body and mind.
Classification: LCC RM666.A68 Y68 2017 (print) | LCC RM666.A68 (ebook) | DDC 615.3/219—dc23
LC record available at https://lccn.loc.gov/2016037295

Llewellyn Worldwide Ltd. does not participate in, endorse, or have any authority or responsibility concerning private business transactions between our authors and the public.

All mail addressed to the author is forwarded, but the publisher cannot, unless specifically instructed by the author, give out an address or phone number.

Any Internet references contained in this work are current at publication time, but the publisher cannot guarantee that a specific location will continue to be maintained. Please refer to the publisher's website for links to authors' websites and other sources.

Llewellyn Publications
A Division of Llewellyn Worldwide Ltd.
2143 Wooddale Drive
Woodbury, MN 55125-2989
www.llewellyn.com

Printed in the United States of America

Contents

Part Two: The Healing Palette of 50 Essential Oils

Part Three: Additional Uses

Disclaimer

I believe there is great value in using essential oils for healing the mind, body, and spirit. Essential oils have historically proven healing properties and therapeutic value. However, you should not substitute the ideas and methods in this book for traditional medical care. Seek advice from your physician for your conditions and use this book with common sense.

The information is presented for educational purposes only and is not intended to diagnose or prescribe for any medical or psychological condition, nor to prevent, treat, mitigate, or cure such conditions. The information herein is not intended as medical advice but rather a sharing of knowledge and information based on research and experience.

Each body reacts differently to natural products and essential oils. One person may have great results with an oil and another may present an allergic reaction. Essential oils are potent and must be used with caution. Always do a patch test on your skin and a gentle smell test to make sure you are using an essential oil that is compatible with your unique chemistry. The bottom line of advice is to do your research and always dilute essential oils before using them, especially with children, as they can have stronger reactions than adults.

Acknowledgments

My first thank-you must go to the godmother of this book, my incredible agent Lisa Hagan. Not only did she have faith in essential oils, she also had faith in me and suggested I write this book. Without her this tome would not exist. Thank you so much Lisa of Lisa Hagan Literary and Lisa Hagan Books. My gratitude is deeper than the ocean.

My second bent-knee curtsey of gratitude goes to Marlene Morris, who read and proofed every word and smoothed every paragraph that may have had a ragged edge or a dangling participle. I share this book with her and am profoundly beholden to her for her patience, unfaltering confidence, cheerleading abilities, and her magnificent show of support.

The third pillar of this three-legged stool is Lisa Tenzin-Dolma, who not only has earned my respect and admiration as an author but also my undying gratitude for her time and effort. She proofread and corrected this book so I could hand it over to my publisher with pride and fewer typos.

Special thanks go to Beth Wareham for her advice, support, and scholarly contributions in the making of this tome. She was a delight to work with!

Lastly, I want to especially thank the very talented and dedicated Registered Aroma Therapist Kelly Holland Azzaro, who is also a Certified Clinical Aromatherapy Practitioner, Certified Bach Flower Practitioner, and a Licensed Massage Therapist. Her hours of help and clarification with the content of this book were out-of-this-world generous and have made it a better book by far.

Introduction

Did essential oils find you, or did you find them? I ask only because the world works in mysterious ways sometimes and you could be on the verge of changing your entire life by learning more about essential oils, their healing properties, and how they can enrich your life.

Obviously something has piqued your interest and drawn you to explore essential oils. Are you just curious? Did you read an article about essential oils and think they sounded interesting? Perhaps a massage therapist dropped some fragrant essences into your massage oil and you can't get the scent out of your mind. In the end, it doesn't matter how you got here, just that you did.

If this is your first foray into essential oils, let me be the first to welcome you into this enchanting world of fragrance, healing, and natural resources. The information in this book will help you learn about the oils, their properties, safe usage, and it will give you a basis for building your own relationship with them. If you allow them to, essential oils will transport you into a brand new world of aromatic sense awakening, physical healing, and natural delights.

For decades I worked up through the ranks in the television industry until I was seasoned enough to produce and direct shows. I observed colleagues crack under the pressure of the long hours and sometimes unhealthy working conditions. One excellent stage manager dropped dead on a set during rehearsal. His heart exploded from the coffee and caffeine he had been using to sustain his energy. I watched stars and crew become addicted to drugs, alcohol, and cigarettes, and that catapulted me toward a healing mission. I didn't want to succumb to the temptations or harm myself. I also wanted to help others beat their issues and choose health over gradual physical erosion.

1

This inclination led me to earn a doctorate in Clinical Hypnotherapy, a doctorate in Natural Healing, and the title of Naturopathic Doctor as a third credential. I have taken many courses in health, healing, biofeedback, past-life regression, Chinese Medicine, and I have traveled to all parts of the world to study under healers and teachers worldwide. I was a licensed general aviation pilot by the age of eighteen, so I'd like to think the view from above enlarged my perspective and appreciation of all aspects of human, plant, mineral, and animal life.

I have studied and written about the healing and vibration energy of Bach Flowers, visited the home and gardens of Dr. Bach in England, and have been participating in the world of essential oils along the way. In my practice, I consult with people who want to change their lifestyle, prolong their lives, and use as many natural products as possible in the process. The list includes weight loss, smoking cessation, addiction therapy, as well as the healing of physical conditions and chronic issues. I choose the appropriate therapy from a wide list of available therapies for my clients based on their needs and preferences.

In preparation for writing this book I took many classes over the course of my three decades of study, visited many websites, attended lectures, and had in-depth conversations with importers, distributors, healers, and Aromatherapists. Sharing the wealth of knowledge from various branches of the essential oil community has been an ongoing honor and privilege.

This book should give you plenty of information about essential oils by passing on what I have learned, describing what they are, what they do, how they work, and how you can use them to enhance your life. The more you know about essential oils, the better they will serve you.

I have grouped the information in the very same way I learned about essential oils: one by one. There is quite a lot to learn and absorb, but I think you'll feel comfortable walking the path I have patterned after my own learning curve.

Part 1 of the book starts as an orientation into this new world and chapter one tells you what the oils are, how they are processed, and provides you with some historical background on essential oils throughout the centuries; in some instances, as far back as five thousand years.

Chapter 2 explains how essential oils work on our bodies and what we can expect to see and experience. In chapter three we discuss the essence of healing and what characterizes the act of healing and why we actually do heal. Chapter four addresses your personal part in the process and asks you, "How will you approach healing with essential oils?" There are several choices for your approach, and you will choose what suits your thinking.

Please read chapters five and six before you go on a purchasing spree. You'll enjoy knowing more about which essential oils to buy as a starting line-up, which essential oils to avoid, which oils combine best together, and suggestions of various carrier oils in which to blend them.

Part two begins with chapters seven through ten and covers the properties, details, and uses for each of the fifty essential oils I favor. This comprehensive study of each oil provides you with a private course that enables you to build a mental library about the oils so you can begin to work wonders.

In part three, as your reward for studying so hard and mastering fifty essential oils, chapter eleven explains how you can use the oils for healing emotions. Chapter twelve discusses how past civilizations have used essential oils throughout history and why they called them sacred. They have become sacred to me too.

Chapter thirteen outlines four alternative methods for using essential oils. You can select from information about chakra healing, the Chinese Five Element system, astrology, and learn how to use charms and talismans for healing. Chapter fourteen is a collection of some of my favorite recipes I have created, discovered, adapted, and used in my own healing practice over the years. (For men and women, the WOW Cream recipe is a skin changer!)

You will uncover a wealth of knowledge about essential oils in these pages and as you experiment with them, you will very likely find yourself falling in love with them as I have. One at a time I learned about each essence and tested them in many different ways for a myriad of purposes. After a short while, I found that I couldn't imagine life without them. Essential oils quickly became irreplaceable members of my extended family. I even travel with them. They even turn my hotel room into a tranquil paradise for adequate rest and recovery from jet lag.

I reflect back to a time when I didn't know about or use essential oils. Life had a different quality back then. I reached automatically for remedies and OTC products that covered up but did not heal my condition. I feel so much better and am happier now because I have studied and incorporated these precious and sacred essences into my life for personal healing on all levels.

If I feel a cold coming on, I'll diffuse a blend of citrus and tea tree or eucalyptus essential oils. For stomach or travel issues, I find peppermint or ginger essential oils will help alleviate discomfort. Bergamot and melissa are my go-to essential oils when I need to be calm for an appointment or interview. Neroli essential oil cheers me up on dark days, and lemon essential oil puts a spring in my step. Ylang-ylang takes care of most impatience and helps me breathe deeper. These essential oils, and many more, are my pals and healing friends. We walk life's path together.

Essential oils of all types continue to bring me new gifts and surprises every day. They are amazing in their properties and what they have to offer us. I believe we are just beginning to realize that they are way ahead of us, and we are the ones who have all the catching up to do.

In closing I want to extend a warm invitation to you to join me on this journey that will launch you on an amazing expedition into the world of essential oils. May it be a glorious excursion.

PART ONE

Basics

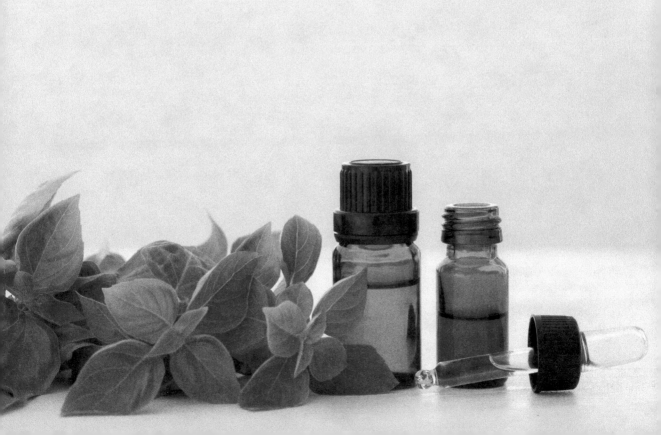

ONE

Essential Oils: What They Are

Essential oils have been, and are to me, many things: they are healers because they assist the body in repairing itself; they are holistic because they involve the whole person, taking into account mental and social factors, as well as physical symptoms; they are sacred because they come from the deepest and richest part of the plant kingdom and have been in use for more than five thousand years. They are natural because they originate from the global ecosystem; they are valuable because they are noninvasive and do not bombard the body with anything artificial or contain human-made chemical properties; they are complementary to human life because they raise the whole person while they help heal; they are considered divine and miraculous by many because they are simple, potent—and some would even say magical—in their uses and effects.

Essential oils are common healing gifts from plants in liquid form. They are easy to use, convenient, portable, charming and fragrant. Essential oils come from the very heart and soul of the plant kingdom. They are green (nonpolluting); deemed natural because they are extracted from the flowers, stems, and roots of living plants; and they are holistic because they affect the whole person as a cohesive unit.

An essential oil is an oil made from a plant or tree that smells like that plant or tree. Essential oils are also called *ethereal oils, volatile oils, aetherolea,* or simply as the "oil of" the plant from which it is extracted. An oil is "essential" in the sense that it contains the characteristic fragrance and properties of the plant that it is taken from.[1]

---

1   Definition of essential oil. info47051.wix.com/aromatherapist#!essential-oil-facts/vyo0v.

7

An essential oil is typically obtained through an advanced process of distillation, expression or solvent extraction.

Distillation

As an example, lavender, peppermint, tea tree, and eucalyptus essential oils are distilled. Raw materials such as seeds flowers, bark, leaves, wood, roots, or the peel of the plant are placed in an alembic still. The word *alembic* means something that refines. For this process, two vessels are connected together by a tube.

One side is heated to produce a vapor that rises as steam then condenses and cools which causes it to run down the connecting tube into the adjacent vessel. Moonshine is made in the same way.

Fascinatingly, the invention of the alembic still is attributed to Cleopatra the alchemist (not the infamous queen of the Nile), who is said to have invented it in the third century.[2] Most oils that are distilled use this single distilling process.

Expression

Generally citrus peel oils are cold-pressed, as is olive oil. Cold-pressing refers to the juicing or pressing process of fruit or vegetables occurring at lower temperatures, thereby preserving more of the original taste, flavor, and nutrients of the original fruit, plant, or vegetable.

Because there is a great deal of oil in citrus peel, citrus oils are more plentiful and less expensive than other essential oils. Well before the invention of the distillation process, all essential oils were extracted by the method of pressing.

Solvent Extraction

Most flowers and buds are extremely delicate and can easily be damaged by the extreme temperatures of steam distillation, so a solvent called a *concrete* is added to separate and remove the oils. A concrete is a mixture of essential oil, waxes, resins, and other oil-soluble plant material. Ethyl alcohol is used in the final process to extract the scent of the oil from the concrete, leaving the chemicals behind.

---

2   Stanton J. Linden, ed., *The Alchemy Reader: From Hermes Trismegistus to Isaac Newton* (New York: Cambridge University Press), 44.

Absolutes

Essential oils and absolutes differ from each other because the absolute contains more coloring, plant waxes, and plant matter; essential oils contain only the oil portion of the plant. Absolutes are used in perfumes more frequently because they are extracted using chemicals like hexane and ethyl alcohol and do contain a small percentage of left over alcohol. Absolutes are highly concentrated aromatic oils extracted from plants and with chemical residue, so are not generally used therapeutically.

CO_2 Extracts

Carbon dioxide gas under pressure is the method used for extracting plant matter. These extracts are obtained using different pressures: *total* means high pressure and *select* means lower pressure in a lower temperature setting. Total extracts contain more of the plant itself and therefore deliver more of the plant's properties than what essential oils provide. CO_2 extracts are used in food, body care, and herbal applications as well as aromatherapy and natural perfumes because they have the purest and truest fragrance of the plant. This is a relatively new method of extraction and the most expensive.

Organic Extracts

Another method for extraction involves organic solvents and alcohol to leach the scent out of plants and flowers/blossoms. This method keeps the fragrances vibrant and provides potent aromatic essences for perfumers, Aromatherapists, and healers.

Hydrosols

Hydrosols are essentially flower waters and are the by-product of the process of steam distilling plant matter. They resemble essential oils but are highly diluted liquids. They are suitable for use in situations where an essential oil might be deemed too potent. They are used in skin care products, as air purifiers, and for body sprays.

Historical Uses of Essential Oils

Essential oils have historically been treated as sacred and date back to a time even before the Egyptians. The ancient Chinese treated mania, depression, and anxiety with essential oils for a thousand years before the pharaohs came to power. Ancient Babylonians perfumed their bodies and mortar for their buildings with essential oils. They adopted the practice from the ancient Vedic Indians who built temples and palaces made from sandalwood to radiate intoxicating aromas for spiritual purposes.

Queen Cleopatra (not the alchemist) seduced her Roman lovers by aromatizing the sails of her ships before launching out onto the Nile to greet them. She wrapped herself in fine linens soaked in fragrant oils, making herself an irresistible catch to some world-famous rulers.

The Egyptians were obsessed with the afterlife and wanted to make sure they had enough food, riches, and sacred oils entombed with them as they crossed the bridge between human life and immortality. Extracting essential oils from plants was a highly-guarded secret by temple hierarchy because the Egyptians revered essential oils and believed them to be healing and sacred. When King Tut's tomb was opened in 1922, 350 liters of essential oils meticulously preserved in alabaster jars were discovered. Waxes made from plant products sealed the containers leaving the oils in impeccable condition for centuries. Even the scent was still detectable three thousand years later and recipes for incenses and oils were found carved on the temple pillar at Edfu, along the Nile.

In the same company as the Babylonians and the Chinese, the Egyptians were among the first people to extensively make use of aromatherapy and aromatic herbs. These herbs were used in religious practices and cosmetics as well as for healing and medicinal purposes. The Egyptians used essential oils in their daily lives to maintain health, for personal hygiene, to lift emotions, and as offerings to their gods. They did not segregate essential oils used for cosmetic purposes (perfumes) from those used for medicinal or spiritual purposes. They were one and the same.

When someone became ill in ancient Egypt, they went to a priest or priestess who selected and administered the appropriate essential oil remedy to relieve the condition, pain, or illness. The Egyptians believed that using such a spiritual or emotional remedy could heal physical problems. They were so smart that they even invented what we know as modern surgical procedures using handcrafted metal instruments for brain and internal organ surgery.

The embalming process called for several essential oils used for their preservation abilities and aroma. Essential oil distillation pots have been found at Tepe Gawra, near the ancient site of Nineveh, dating back to circa 3500 BCE.[3]

Among the oldest healing oils that have been used since antiquity are cassia, cinnamon, frankincense, galbanum, myrrh, and spikenard. The Bible speaks of fourteen sacred and healing oils: calamus, cassia, cedarwood, cinnamon, cypress, fir, frankincense, galbanum, hyssop, juniper, myrrh, myrtle, pine, and spikenard.[4]

In ancient times the Egyptians bought shiploads of resins from the Phoenicians and used them for perfume, salves, incense, insect repellent, and for wounds and sores. Myrrh oil made the skin young again, while frankincense was burned, turned into charcoal, and ground into the heavy kohl eyeliner Egyptian women so famously wore. Murals decorating the walls of a temple dedicated to Queen Hatshepsut depicted sacks of frankincense and saplings of myrrh trees in the painting. Hatshepsut ruled Egypt for two decades circa 480 BCE.[5]

Kyphi was the main scent of Egyptian temples. A daily temple ritual consisted of burning frankincense in the morning, myrrh at midday, and kyphi at night.[6]

The beliefs and wisdom of the Egyptian physicians and healers were carried to Greece by ancient mariners and travelers. The most well-known physician of that time, Hippocrates (c. 460–377 BCE), based his practice on treating the patient holistically. He once said that *natural forces within us are the true healers of disease,* a principle in which he firmly believed and taught.[7]

---

3   Brian Peasnall and Mitchell S. Rothman, "One of Iraq's Earliest Towns," Expedition, vol. 45, no. 3, University of Pennsylvania Museum, www.penn.museum/documents/publications /expedition/PDFs/45–3/One%20of%20Iraq.pdf.

4   "Oils of the Bible" www.essential-oil-mama.com/essential-oils-of-the-bible.html.

5   Jennie Cohen, "A Wise Man's Cure: Frankincense and Myrhh" www.history.com/news /a-wise-mans-cure-frankincense-and-myrrh.

6   Victor Loret, "Le kyphi, parfum sacré des anciens égyptiens," *Asiatique 10 (juillet-août):* 1887, 76–132.

7   www.brainyquote.com/quotes/quotes/h/hippocrate133221.html.

Often he included aromatherapy massage as part of his treatments. He is credited with changing the way medicine was viewed, and he used herbal plants and essential oils as part of his healing theory and protocol.

The Romans learned about the ancient oils (and plants) from the Greeks. They got on the hygiene bandwagon and referred to them as secrets of health. They also practiced aromatherapy using the power of fragrances to soothe and heal.

After the Roman Empire collapsed, Europe fell into the Dark Ages, and space was provided for Arabian scholars and physicians to emerge with their sophistication of and reverence for essential oils. Known primarily for their use in incense and ancient rituals, frankincense and myrrh also demonstrated antiseptic and anti-inflammatory properties and were used as effective remedies for everything including leprosy and toothaches. International teacher Alain Touwaide, historian and founder of the Institute for the Preservation of Medical Traditions and researcher for the Smithsonian writes:

> We have textual and also archaeological evidence that both frankincense and
> myrrh were used as medicinal substances in antiquity.[8]

Frankincense was used in traditional Chinese medicine as early as 500 BCE. The Chinese and Indian cultures used many essential oils for healing, deity worship, during ritual consecrations, and ceremonies honoring their ancestors.

Both frankincense and myrrh have a five-thousand-year old history of being traded in the Middle East and North Africa.[9] It is believed that the Babylonians and Assyrians burned them for religious ceremonies. The Persian physician Avicenna (980–1037 CE) is assigned the accolade for experimenting with and perfecting the distillation process of essential oils following Cleopatra the Alchemist's invention of the alembic still.

Moving into the Dark Ages (500 CE to 1000 CE) we find that cloistered monks grew magnificent gardens of healing plants and herbs and used them for the care and cure of ill villagers. In those darkest of days, folk medicine and the use of herbal remedies normally lead to the persecution and death of those healers and practitioners who were unceremoni-

---

8   Jennie Cohen, "A Wise Man's Cure: Frankincense and Myrrh," www.history.com/news/a-wise
     -mans-cure-frankincense-and-myrrh.

9   Ibid.

ously accused of being witches and using potions. The clever monks were able to preserve the knowledge and the practice of herbal medicine because they were revered and deemed holy, thereby placing them above the law or persecution from church authorities.

While personal cleanliness was not practiced as a rule in thirteenth- and fourteenth-century medieval Europe, essential oils were very popular. The Roman Church had admonished its followers that bathing was sinful, so people turned to aromatics to keep stench at bay and avoid the *sin* of bathing, for which punishment was doled out. Essential oils have antibacterial and pesticidal properties that under the guise of stench abatement, rendered many threatening germs harmless. We now know that the lack of sanitation and bathing contributed to the spread of plagues.

Many historical accounts tell us that the four thieves who robbed bubonic plague victims in the fifteenth century and did not catch the illness were actually merchant spice traders and perfumers who bathed in aromatic herbal infused vinegar with balsam, cinnamon, clove, frankincense, pine, and rosemary. As a result of the antibacterial qualities of these mixtures they were subsequently, and a tad mysteriously, rendered immune to the plague. That recipe is still in circulation today.

During the Renaissance there was a modest return to the holistic treatment of illness and disease. The noted physician Paracelsus (Phillipus Aureolus Theophrastus Bombastus von Hohenheim, 1493–1541) explored the beliefs and practices of folk medicine and included its wisdom and value in his healing methods. His claim to fame was a cure for leprosy using herbal remedies.

The term "aromatherapy" based on the use of essential oils was coined by the French chemist and perfumer Rene Maurice Gattefossé in 1937. He had been transformed into a die-hard believer in 1910, when late one night in his laboratory he burnt his hand rather seriously and developed gas gangrene. The closest available compound was pure, undiluted lavender oil. In his own words, according to Robert Tisserand who translated it from French:

Just one rinse with lavender essence stopped "the gasification of the tissue. Healing began the next day (July 1910)."[10]

---

10 René Maurice Gattefossé and Robert Tisserand, ed. *Gattefossé's Aromatherapy: The First Book on Aromatherapy* (London: Random House, 1987), 87.

Tisserand contends that using lavender essential oil as a remedy was intentional and the healing was a remarkable moment for the field of "Aroma Therapy," a term Gattefossé coined in his 1937 book *Aromatherapie*.[11]

In further experiments, Gattefossé discovered that even small amounts of essential oils, readily absorbed by the body, can interact with bodily chemistry depending on how they are applied. His nocturnal misfortune opened the door for a whole new era of his exploration into the healing benefits of essential oils.

During the second World War, Dr. Jean Valnet used essential oils with great success to treat injured soldiers. He based his treatments on the research of his predecessor, Rene Gattefossé. In further experiments, Valnet found that he was able to cure longterm psychiatric patients by administering essential oils with almost immediate results. In 1964, Dr. Valnet wrote:

It is conceivable that the day will come when the true therapeutic value of natural substances will be given proper recognition.[12]

On the heels of WWII, Marguerite Maury, an Austrian-born biochemist, began experimenting with diluting essential oils in a vegetable-based carrier oil to use them as massage therapy for her clients in the 1950s. We are not sure if this began as a matter of thrift, or if she wanted to explore the same dilution techniques that homeopathy employs.

First she mixed her oils, and then applied the diluted oils along the spinal column specifically targeting the nerve endings on her client's back according to a Tibetan technique she had learned. Ms. Maury is credited as being the first person to use individual preparations and blends of essential oils to suit the specific needs of the person being massaged based solely on their personality and physical needs she skillfully assessed beforehand.

During the late 1970s and early 80s, the use of essential oils and aromatherapy rose in popularity and became a major component of alternative and holistic therapeutic

---

11   "Gatefossé's Burn," roberttisserand.com/2011/04/gattefosses-burn/.

12   Jean Valnet, *The Practice of Aromatherapy* (Richmond, VT: Healing Arts Press, 1982), 89.

treatment. Essential oils are now extremely popular worldwide; it is estimated that sales are in the billions worldwide.[13]

Western medicine has slowly begun to validate their healing properties. At the French Police Toxicology Laboratory, Professor Griffon, director, set out to test the anti-septic effects of specifically chosen essential oils. He blended pine, thyme, peppermint, lavender, rosemary, clove, and cinnamon essential oils. He placed several petri dishes about six inches above the floor. He allowed the dishes to collect microbes for a period of twenty-four hours. The next day, he tested them again and found they contained 210 colonies of microbes including several varieties of molds and staphylococci. He added his prepared blend of essential oils to the dishes. Within thirty minutes, all of the potentially harmful, disease-causing molds and staphylococci were destroyed.[14]

Peppermint has been shown to reduce nausea for pregnant women during labor. In another study, neroli essential oil helped reduce blood pressure and pre-procedure anxiety among people undergoing a colonoscopy.[15]

These and so many more ongoing clinical studies will continue to help us bring ancient knowledge together with modern treatments. Each belief system and practice has merit and value. We have the superb option of choosing the most effective and least harmful remedies for our intricate physical systems.

The best news is that essential oils are available to everyone for purposes of their choosing, whether it be physical healing, developing mental clarity, or seeking an emotional lift. They are natural gifts eagerly waiting to help improve our daily lives.

---

13   "The Global Essential Oil Trade," www.crnm.org/index.php?option=com_docman&task=doc
      _view&gid=106&tmpl=component&format=raw&Itemid=113. *Global Oil Trade* volume 25,
      Sept/Oct 2007.

14   "Essential Oils," hopewelloils.com/medicinal-value.php.

15   Steve Erlich, NMD, "Aromatherapy," umm.edu/health/medical/altmed/treatment
      /aromatherapy#ixzz3fX0u9194.

TWO

Essential Oils: How They Work

Researchers are not entirely clear how aromatherapy works. According to studies at the University of Maryland Medical Center, experts believe the sense of smell may play a key role because this important sense is directly linked to the emotions. When you inhale an aroma the molecules gain access to a central part of your brain called the amygdala. This area is part of the limbic system and was at one time known as the "smell brain." The scent receptors in your nose communicate with specific parts of your brain (the amygdala and the hippocampus) that serve as warehouses for emotions and memories. When you breathe in essential oil molecules, some researchers believe they stimulate these parts of your brain and influence physical, emotional, and mental health. For example, scientists believe lavender stimulates the activity of brain cells in the amygdala similar to the way some sedative medications like Ativan and Valium work.[16] Other researchers believe molecules from essential oils interact in the blood with hormones or enzymes.[17] Healing and improvement occurs at the molecular and cellular level in the human body. That's the only thing we know for sure.

---

16   Erhlich NMD, Steve, "Lavender," University of Maryland Medical Center, http://umm.edu/health/medical/altmed/herb/lavender accessed 10/2/2015

17   Erhlich, "Aromatherapy."

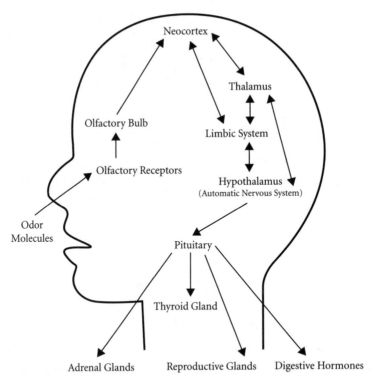

The Limbic System: "smell brain"

Besides being a center of scent receptors, the limbic system is the storehouse for all of our past emotional responses.[18] It is located deep within the medial temporal lobe of the brain and includes the hippocampus, amygdala, cingulate gyrus, thalamus, hypothalamus, epithalamus, the mammillary body, and other organs, many of which are of particular relevance to the processing of memory.[19] The result is that we have both a past and present sense memory available to us at all times. Helen Keller said:

> Smell is a potent wizard that transports us across thousands of miles and all the years we have lived.[20]

---

18   "Parts of the Brain," www.human-memory.net/brain_parts.html.

19   Ibid.

20   Helen Keller, attr. thinkexist.com/quotation/smell_is_a_potent_wizard_that_transports _you/209065.html.

Fragrance has been successfully used to enhance and create positive emotions. It can also clear emotional negativity or blockages that may have been created by past experiences and lodged in the memory. The removal of negative emotional thoughts or recollections and the replacement of them with positive ideas facilitates the healing process. This is the goal of healing with aromatherapy: to remove what doesn't serve us and replace it with something that does.

Besides smelling and inhaling the fragrance of essential oils, we can apply them and in some circumstances (only under the supervision of a certified Aromatherapist), ingest some of them. The body easily metabolizes the natural molecules of essential oils because they come from plant matter. Our bodies were designed to handle and manage them quite efficiently and naturally.

Certain essential oils are matched with specific receptors in the brain. It's like finding the right key to open a lock. When an essential oil molecule finds the receptor site it was designed to fit, it passes on its healing information to the cell. When the message has been delivered the essential oil heads to the liver and the kidneys and moves out of the body. Its benefits have been conveyed and its job is complete and it doesn't need to hang around for applause. Regardless of whether the essential oil is used as an application, a bath, a steam inhalation, a compress, in a diffuser, or by other various methods, it connects at the molecular level with the body and gets straight to work.

By contrast, the unnatural molecules of man-made drugs can attach themselves to various tissues and disrupt normal functions for years. The body must figure out what to do with the residuals after the pharmaceuticals have served their purpose. As visitors who never quite leave, they can affect bodily functions, hormonal balances, blood circulation, and even the mind. When you reach your golden years, you will still be able to find traces lingering in your body from prescription drugs you took as a child.[21]

Dr. Andrew Weil frequently uses the image of a polluted river to describe the buildup of toxins or disease in the body. To a point, the body is designed to deal with and excrete certain toxic properties, but it can reach a saturation point and become polluted from excessive toxic substances. Only when the toxins are removed can the body (river) return to normal homeostasis. If the organs of the body cannot stay ahead of eliminating

---

21   Christina Dye, "Drugs and the Body: How Drugs Work," www.doitnow.org/pages/223.html.

toxins or are overburdened by the quantity, toxic substances stay in the waste-holding area of the body (usually fatty tissue, including the brain) where they can hang out for years, or even a lifetime, upsetting normal body functions for as long as they linger. And we've all had the experience of a guest who overstays their welcome, haven't we?

Most natural and nontoxic organic substances such as essential oils are easily eliminated by the body when their usefulness runs its course.

They enter, they perform, and then they leave without causing harm or side effects. (There are a few exceptions to this rule we will cover in the section on safety.)[22]

Whereas many drugs can depress the immune system, essential oils can strengthen it. Antibiotics attack invasive bacteria indiscriminately, killing both the good and the bad. Essential oils assail only the harmful bacteria, allowing the body's friendly flora to flourish and helping prevent cancer, diabetes, and other inflammatory diseases.[23]

After learning how our bodies process substances, I try to minimize the use of pharmaceutical drugs by considering what essential oils can offer.

I seldom reach for an aspirin to cure a headache, instead using helichrysum, peppermint, or even lemon essential oil diluted. Sometimes I rub the mixture between my palms and sniff the essential oil mix for fast relief.

Other times I diffuse a blend of the above adding eucalyptus to fill the room and surround myself with the headache relief mist. I always begin with a gentle and natural approach. If I can't relieve my symptoms, I call my physician for an appointment.

I encourage everyone to look a bit deeper, explore other options—that have been around for centuries—and make assessments based on holistic principles.

Ask: "What is best for my mind, body, and soul as a unit?" When we take an active interest in our personal health choices and have confidence that we *do* know a lot more intuitively than we give ourselves credit for, we begin the process of healing from the inside out.

---

22   David Stewart, "Why Essential Oils Heal and Drugs Don't," healthimpactnews.com/2013 /why-essential-oils-heal-and-drugs-dont/.

23   Emma Inness, "Is Gut Bacteria the Secret to Long Life?" www.dailymail.co.uk/health /article-2541272/Is-gut-bacteria-secret-LONG-LIFE-Friendly-flora-reduces-inflammation -prevents-disease-claims-study.html.

Essential oils are one of the many options we have for solving health challenges. They have properties that help us by balancing the body and addressing the *causes* of disease at the cellular level.

When essential oils are properly applied they work toward the restoration of cooperative bodily functions. When multiple systems become involved in fixing the problem, they work in partnership with each other to heal. This is the perfect kind of healing committee we want working on our behalf.

Essential oils come from plants that are rooted in the earth. As such, they have a different vibration than humans do. Current research is exploring the electrical frequency of the human body and how we can cure through vibrations of sound, light, and the body's own frequency.

A radiologist from Stockholm, Sweden, Bjorn Nordenstrom, discovered in the early 1980s that by putting an electrode inside a tumor and running a milliamp of direct current through the electrode, he could dissolve a cancer tumor and stop its growth.[24]

He also found that the human body had electropositive and electronegative energy fields. Engineer and author Debbie Takara Shelor writes:

> The highest frequency emotion is enthusiasm. Love and joy also fall into this category. This is followed by pain (emotional or physical) which is followed by anger. The next lower frequency emotion is fear, which is followed by grief. Below grief is apathy. Finally, the lowest frequency emotion is unconsciousness (meaning it is so awful we have completely blocked out those situations from our lives). If we are experiencing anything less than enthusiasm in any area of our life, we have lowered our frequency and are running the risk of disease. In order to be healthy, people must increase their frequency.[25]

---

24 Dr. Nordenstrom was a member of the Nobel Prize committee in Medicine and Physics and was awarded the International Scientific and Technological Cooperation Award by the People's Republic of China because of his work on tumor regression.

25 Debbie Takara Shelor, "What is Vibrational Medicine or Energy Healing?" www.magnificentu .com/vibrational-medicine-energy-healing.

Tainio Technology, an independent division of Eastern State University in Cheny, Washington, conducted studies in 1992 that reinforced the findings of earlier researchers.[26]

Tainio and colleagues discovered through frequency testing that when a person's frequency drops below the optimum healthy range, the immune system is compromised. Below is a sample of their findings:

- Human cells can start to change (mutate) when their frequency drops below 62 MHz.

- 58 MHz is the frequency noted in the body when you get a cold or the flu.

- *Candida* can be recognized when a body presents a vibration at 55 MHz.

- 52 MHz is the frequency of a body when the Epstein-Barr virus is present.

- 42 MHz is the frequency of a body that allows cancer cells to flourish.

- When the frequency of the body drops to 20 MHz the death process commences.[27]

Tainio also provided speculation that "even thoughts and feelings have a vibratory quality that forms a measurable frequency" and a negative mental state can lower a person's frequency by 10–12 MHz.[28] Although biologist Bruce Tainio died in 2009, his work for seeds and agriculture continues through his company.

The properties of essential oils are excellent natural choices we can use to rebalance and encourage the innate healing capabilities of the body.

Purposed to heal, they go right to the source and begin work. Incorporated as part of a wellness program, they can sustain the body, supporting health and promoting physical harmony.

---

26 "Vibrational Frequency and the Subtle Energy of Essential Oils," www.biospiritual-energy-healing.com/vibrational-frequency.html.

27 Ibid.

28 Ibid.

THREE

How We Heal

We have all watched a flesh wound heal and certainly appreciate our body's ability to repair and restore a nasty mishap caused by a sharp knife or a rusty nail. If we stop to think about it, it's an amazing inter-functional process of cell replacement, blood clotting, and the unseen forces at work that repair the damage. But what do we really know about how healing happens or why it even occurs? We take it for granted that we will heal. Who or what tells the body to heal? Who or what gives the instructions? And who or what follows them?

The population is divided on the subject of healing. Some believe only medical doctors can achieve it, prescribe it, or make it occur. Others believe healing and cures can be achieved through complementary and alternative methods that involve the participation of the totality of a person and not just the parts.

Still unanswered is the ever-present question: Why does one person heal yet another does not? Can the mysterious healing process be explained by the body of knowledge we call "science" or should we turn to something like "art" for answers?

Science follows facts, collects data, studies multiple examples or cases, and then offers a conclusion or diagnosis. Art, on the other hand, is the free expression of the creative mind, spirit, inspiration, and emotions. Art begins with an idea and incorporates tools to turn that idea into something that can be seen or shared. If we consider the process of healing as an art, rather than a science, we invite invisible creative forces to enlighten our expression and unleash our imagination. This approach allows us to go beyond the mundane and access previously undiscovered possibilities for healing. The artistic way of healing inspires the creative genius within each one of us and fosters cooperation of the mind (beliefs), the body (the natural healer), and the spirit (courage and optimism). This combination of elements causes healing to occur.

When we get down to the nitty-gritty of how healing happens, we uncover what Bruce Lipton suggests:

There's a force moving within us, a biological imperative to survive and avoid death.[29]

That force is so strong that it always seeks a cure, always wants to heal, and has a built-in GPS for recovery and wellness. The body's natural programming is to heal itself. It gets off track when we interfere with its natural programming and direction by polluting it with too many chemicals or over-processed foods. Another thing we do know about healing is that it is, by its very nature, cooperative. The act of healing involves many systems, many parts of the body and is most successful when the mind and the spirit join hands and get behind the process. We are served best when we use the more creative and inspired art of healing approach that includes using all the tools at our disposal, both natural and man-made.

Naturopathic doctors use principles that are based on observations of how a disease behaves and manifests in the body as well as clinical scientific data and research. Naturopaths consider the underlying emotions and the mental state, and they use natural products as both an art and science for diagnosis and healing of a client. They evaluate all the layers of the person and how the condition may have developed in the first place. They try to find the real cause of the condition that may elude some health practitioners. Naturopaths seek to release a person's inner healer.

With this knowledge we are free to use many people and many things for healing including medical doctors, alternative therapy healers, and a host of other disciplines, techniques, and products. Healing can occur from unexpected sources.

Consider for a moment what *Power Versus Force* author David Hawkins writes:

Medicine has forgotten that it was an art and that science was merely a tool of that art.[30]

---

29   Bruce Lipton, www.BruceLipton.com.

30   David Hawkins, MD, PhD, *Power Versus Force* (Carlsbad, CA: Hay House, 2014), 28.

If you are willing to consider healing more as an art rather than only a science, imagine the new horizons that are open to you! Possibilities are widened and there are unlimited opportunities to explore healing from myriad angles. We can look to nature, we can access eastern and western medicine, we can participate in rituals, and we can align our minds and hearts with the cosmic power held in the moon, the stars, the sun, and the planets. We can attune our bodies to the four directions, to the meridians described in Chinese medicine, and to the chakras from the Vedas or other sacred practices. We can partner art and science as our sources for healing.

You might be wondering where we would look if we want to find the hidden power behind healing. Where is the magic in healing? And most importantly, where do we begin?

We can start by looking at the process and practice of the artist as healer. According to the David Hawkins school of thought, if we allow science to supersede the art, we approach the concept of healing in reverse as well. In this backward equation, healing might be considered to be an accident or a by-product of the tool rather than the natural outcome of our artful practices.

Michelangelo was once asked to reveal the secret of his art. He is reported to have replied:

> "I saw the angel in the marble and carved until I set him free."[31] When asked specifically about his masterpiece, *David,* he shrugged, "It's easy. I just chip away anything that isn't *David.*"[32]

When we consider Michelangelo's *David* as a masterpiece of the inner artist, the chisel and the marble become mere tools the artist uses to achieve full artistic expression. If we think and act like an artist when we approach healing, we can look at outside elements as tools, not limitations. Like Michelangelo, we need to understand that the art of healing comes from the wisdom that lives within our true selves and not from outside implements. The tools of science are meant to serve the healing arts, not the other way around. Essential oils are natural tools that we can use to unlock the healing that is already within.

---

31   Michelangelo, attr., www.brainyquote.com/quotes/quotes/m/michelange108779.html.

32   Ibid.

Science as we understand it is only a few hundred years old, pretty young in the historical annals of the world. It has been called a great adventure in that it explores awesome and unknown regions ranging from the human body, to the ancient oak tree, to the stars and beyond.

Some philosophers pit science against art, dubbing science as mortally limited to facts and figures while knighting art as the source of everything magical and the essence of human expression. Jean-Jacques Rousseau criticized the sciences for distancing man from nature and not operating to make people happier.

> "Both [sides] have it wrong," wrote Ray Spangenburg. "Nothing could be more growth oriented or more filled with wonder or more human. Science is constantly evolving, undergoing revolutions, always producing 'new words set to the old music,' and constantly refocusing what has gone before into fresh, new understanding."[33]
>
> Ralph Waldo Emerson wrote, "Science does not know its debt to imagination."[34]

I like his thinking because the day the two worlds figure it out, we'll have a perfect blend of science and art. Healing will no longer be a mystery or a miracle but an everyday occurrence for every human being on earth.

Science and nature can coexist and work hand in hand to improve the human condition. Imagination is a key component to healing and the engine that drives the healing artist forward. It may be invisible, but its potency can be felt around the world. Tapping into both imagination and memory, the mind can picture the body restored, whole, and healed; the body can feel it accomplished. This is the moment of synergy when healing takes root.

The art of healing is analogous to the art of creation. Both are processes of indeterminable length; they can happen in an instant or over the span of an entire lifetime. At

---

33   Ray Spangenburg and Diane Kit Moser, *The Birth of Science: Ancient Times to 1699* (Facts on File, 2004), preface.

34   www.brainyquote.com/quotes/quotes/r/ralphwaldo107616.html

the core of all healing is the act of co-creating with our physical universe, and the same is true for art. Perhaps the art of creation and the creation of art are one and the same; because both require imagination for their outcome. Healing occurs first in the mind of the artist and then travels into the body and spirit of the person being healed.

Let's stay with the concept that healing is an art for a moment—a uniquely individual art wherein the process unfolds differently for each person. What may heal one person may not heal another. The healing artist incorporates knowledge, intuition, and instinct to explore the dimensions of healing and to guide the process to completion. The healing artist uses care and compassion, valuing not only that which is being healed but the very art of healing itself.

Essential oils are extraordinary healers because they work by using the physical properties of the plant essences combined with imagination, creativity, and the heart of the healing artist. The visible and the invisible combine forces to provide the body a way to heal. The body accepts those properties and intentions and sets about the process of self-restoration,something it understands impeccably and innately. As the healing artist, you select an essential oil possessing properties that can relieve a certain complaint, and filled with knowledge and confidence, you administer the oil appropriately.

Mastering the art of healing is like allowing the layers that suppress the inner artist to peel away. As the veils of skepticism or timidity that block our connection to our inner healer are lifted, we are automatically launched into the sacred realm of healer and healing. The art shows up as the definition of healing: "the expression or application of human creative skill and imagination," and healing emerges from that center of our being outwards. From the thought or intention to heal (imagination) comes the process of application/action (the use of essential oils), and the manifestation of the combination of the two which we know to be healing.[35]

When regarded as an art, the process of healing is an open playing field to all people regardless of education, status, race, or creed. Healing is a natural gift and it is the birthright of everyone on earth to enjoy health and restoration. Essential oils provide a gateway to the art of healing, and this book gives you the tools to become a true healing artist.

---

35   Merriam-Webster, www.merriam-webster.com.

FOUR

The Healing Artist's Palette

As I became more comfortable with my journey into the art of healing using essential oils, I learned to appreciate and use them like the dollops of paint on an artist's palette. The more I thought about essential oils being like a selection of colors an artist might use for creating her masterpiece, the more the metaphor clicked into place for me.

I have come to regard essential oils as a color palette in the same way a painter approaches the tools of her art. First you choose a subject, next you select the colors you want to work with and then you greet the blank canvas. With inspiration, many brush strokes and inspired mixing of color and light the masterpiece emerges. Almost like magic, it comes to life on the canvas right before your eyes.

In the world of the painter are the basic or primary colors: red, blue, and yellow. Then there are the secondary colors which are made up of the primary colors blended together: red and yellow combine to make orange, yellow and blue make green, and red plus blue yields purple. When you mix the three primary colors of red, blue, and yellow together, you get a tertiary color. You can continue on ad infinitum mixing primary, secondary, and tertiary colors and produce an unlimited palette with your prolific imagination. So it is with essential oils.

I found that just like the multiple tiers of the color wheel, there are also levels in the process of getting to know the oils, experimenting with them and integrating them into daily life. I have organized the selection of essential oils in levels from beginning and basic to the more complex and rich. Just as an artist can paint a picture using the primary colors of red, blue, and yellow, you can use the first set of twelve essential oils as your primary palette. I chose this first set of twelve based on three criteria: information taught by experts, my own experimentation, and ease of availability and use.

The primary palette contains the building blocks of healing with essential oils. Like the painter's primary colors, they are the basics. They work for you individually or in combination with each other. The primary palette consists of twelve essential oils: lavender, tea tree, rosemary, lemon, bergamot, peppermint, eucalyptus, Roman chamomile, frankincense, sandalwood, thyme, and ylang-ylang.

The secondary palette, another set of twelve wonderful essential oils, offers you greater choices and more flexibility in creating blends for healing, relaxation and general life improvement. This palette selection came about as a result of experimentation, more conditions to heal, and my own sense of adventure. This group increased my kaleidoscope and gave me many more healing options. Since this palette creates deeper colors and a wider range of combinations and possibilities, I was able to create more recipes and have more options for addressing physical and emotional issues. The secondary palette consists of: patchouli, rose, black pepper, clary sage, ginger, orange, helichrysum, vetiver, basil, neroli, marjoram, and yarrow essential oils.

Using the tertiary palette is where it really gets exciting as you gain efficacy with twelve more essential oils and discover how much more you can do with them alone or blended together. This palette provides an even larger range of possibilities for recipes and combinations. The increased possibilities gave me a big enough repertoire to satisfy the needs of my family and clients. As I went along on my healing path I discovered that some, not all, of the qualities and properties were duplicated from the first two levels, but the scent or the effect of the oil was just different enough to merit being in my healing cabinet as an addition or alternative to the twenty-four I had already collected. They are: geranium, melissa, clove bud, spikenard, benzoin, ravensara, cedarwood, cinnamon, lemongrass, palo santo, pink grapefruit, and dill.

This process of adding a layer at a time led me to the final level I call the master's palette. These are the rare and fragrant essential oils and absolutes that are so much fun to work and play with; so rewarding and yet not mandatory for your initial healing kit or work. They are simply the most desirable premium oils in the world and they are for the advanced level.

The master's palette consists of fourteen specialty oils that are more expensive than most but add an element of richness to the previous essential oils palettes. It is as if you are adding real diamonds to the sky when you paint your version of *Starry Night*. The master's palette represents the over-the-top most exotic, potent, and powerful premium essential oils and absolutes in the world. These are the ultimate resources for the healing artist as we go on to create advanced level masterpieces worthy of the aroma museum. (There isn't one yet, but there should be!) The master's palette consists of: champaca, tuberose, coffee flower, frangipani, cannabis flower, agarwood, Bulgarian rose, seaweed, elecampane, Indian sandalwood, carnation, jasmine, blue chamomile, and hops.

The more you use the primary palette of essential oils, the more you will enjoy and be thrilled with the benefits that they bring. Then, in time, you'll want to add even more of them from your secondary palette for use in advanced recipes and applications. By the time you reach the tertiary palette you'll know what you want more of and your instincts will guide you toward a selection of additional essential oils that are perfect for you. As for the master's palette, well, we all have goals and dreams; it may require a savings plan, but there are some luscious premium essential oils and absolutes on this list.

The objective of this book is to provide you with essential oil basics, a handful of ideas for using them, and simple recipes to get you started. I know from my own experience that as I grew in proficiency, I intuitively knew which essential oils I wanted to add to my collection to broaden my spectrum of healing possibilities. Every artist knows what is best for his or her medium. With this information you will be able to expand beyond the basics and use your own essential oil palette and blends to become the healing artist of your own life and that of others.

Once you select the essential oils for your palette the blending, combining, and use of the essential oils is left entirely up to the creative artist in you. The first step is to acquaint yourself with the properties of the oils and then experiment with how you can use them in various aspects of your life. Read about essential oil cautions in the next chapter before you use them for physical healing, burns, cuts, scars, aches, pains, abrasions, and for mental, spiritual, and emotional transformation as well as cleaning and purifying your home.

In the exploration of essential oils there are no hard and fast rules. Nothing limits your resourcefulness when you approach them as healer and artist. You can utilize your essential oils for myriad purposes for the mind, body, and soul.

FIVE

Using Essential Oils

I remember the very first essential oil I bought. It was lavender and I used it in a diffuser ring around a light bulb on my bed table. That was quite a first experience. I had been having trouble sleeping, and as the scent filled the room it somehow lulled my over-active mind to sleep. I was super impressed and grateful for the much-needed rest. One oil led to another, and pretty soon I was creating my own blends for sleep, rest, soul soothing, massage, and a host of other uses.

Every time I found a new essential oil, my life changed for the better. Sometimes it was in a big, dramatic way; other times there was a gentler shift. I was able to alleviate stress headaches with essential oil blends I made. I was able to settle an upset stomach using ginger essential oil and my skin took on a new radiance when I used a creative mixture on my face. Every room in the house has some essential oil in it. The kitchen and bathrooms have disinfecting and air freshening oils; the laundry room has odor-abating and fabric freshening oils; the bedroom has relaxing and sleep-inducing oils, and the living room keeps a collection of seasonally appropriate oils to welcome guests with the smell of the month.

I have to admit my first experiences with essential oils were a bit helter-skelter. I don't recommend the hunt and peck method to anyone. It's a much better idea to spend a few moments reading about the qualities of each essential oil before you acquire it. Sure, you can jump right in and figure it out by yourself as you go along, but with a little more knowledge you'll start with a selection of oils that allows you not only the freedom to experiment but also the joy of immediate success. Please be sure to read the cautions about using each essential oil.

As you become proficient and develop a working knowledge of each essential oil's properties, benefits, and cautions, you'll be able to put it to its best use. The more you know, the richer your rewards will be.

I have also included some esoteric material about each essential oil's ruling planet, gender, and element. You may discover that your use of essential oils expands to include alternative healing methods from the worlds of astrology, chakra balancing, yoga, and other philosophical techniques where this information could be beneficial to you.

There are some important facts you might want to know before working with essential oils. The following are some considerations that suggest areas of caution and safety for using them.

Cautions

Starting out exploring essential oils, you will find a lot of sellers on the Internet (and store shelves) who claim that their oil is the best and better than the next seller. Whose marketing do you believe? The advertising industry, speaking in general and broad terms, is focused on one thing: selling products. As a whole, they are not interested in your well-being, your finances, your healing, or your great-aunt Sally.

They succeed in their mission only when you open your wallet to buy. Keep this in mind so that when you are bombarded with the advertising patter; you'll remember that they are primarily interested in their own gain, not yours. Sure, they want you to be satisfied with your purchase so you'll come back to buy more, but that is as far as their concern goes. Many commercially available oils are mixed with synthetic products.

To protect your own best interests you must take the stance of "buyer beware." There are many conscientious and honest suppliers, makers, and bottlers of essential oils. There are many that have high integrity, and there are some that do not. Below are some clarifications and considerations to keep in mind so you can make informed decisions about the essential oils you buy.

Purity

There are two things to evaluate. The first is whether or not the essential oil is organic. When the plant is farmed it can be grown with pesticides or organically. As the plant material is harvested and refined to make the essential oil, everything becomes more potent as it is reduced to an essence.

Essential oils are highly concentrated. If there is only organic matter to refine, you end up with an organic essence. If it is not farmed organically, there may be chemicals present on the leaves and plant matter that are also reduced in the extraction process (through distillation, expression, solvent, effleurage, or CO_2) and the potency of those toxins is increased during the refining process. In other words, you end up with toxins in the essential oil that have been made stronger by refinement. It's like eating fish that has a high content of mercury. The benefits of eating the fish may be outweighed by the negatives, i.e., the contaminants in the flesh.

According to the National Association for Holistic Aromatherapy (NAHA):

Carbon dioxide extraction has been demonstrated to concentrate from 7 to 53 times more pesticide residues in the final extract. Therefore, it seems pertinent to only use organic plant material for CO_2 extraction.[36] That's just one example.

Like food, a living plant can only be certified as organic if it meets the government standards of organic farming. The USDA National Organic Program (NOP) defines organic as follows:

Organic food is produced by farmers who emphasize the use of renewable resources and the conservation of soil and water to enhance environmental quality for future generations. Organic meat, poultry, eggs, and dairy products come from animals that are given no antibiotics or growth hormones. Organic food is produced without using most conventional pesticides; fertilizers made with synthetic ingredients or sewage sludge; bioengineering; or ionizing radiation. Before a product can be labeled "organic," a government-approved certifier inspects the farm where the food is grown to make sure the farmer is following all the rules necessary to meet USDA organic standards. Companies that handle or process organic food before it gets to your local supermarket or restaurant must be certified, too.

---

36 "How Are Essential Oils Extracted?" www.naha.org/explore-aromatherapy/about-aromatherapy/how-are-essential-oils-extracted.

Essential oils are agricultural products and under the governmental rules what constitutes an organic agricultural product is regulated by agencies such as the Department of Agriculture (USDA) in the USA and the National Organic Program (NOP).[37] In Europe, Japan, Australia, and elsewhere, the certifying programs are similar in that third party agencies regulate what is organically farmed and how the processing facility meets individual government regulation. The actual farms and facilities receive the organic certification, not the product itself, so the products that are grown and processed at certified facilities are what are labeled as certified organic.

If you are importing or purchasing essential oils from Europe, here is what you need to look for:

The US imports organic European products which qualifies for the USDA organic labeling if: (products from) animals are antibiotic-free and pesticide free in the care and feeding of the animal or plant *and* a certificate is issued by a certifying organization which attests to the compliance of the organic prerequisites.[38]

Organic and wild harvested products from Europe may carry the label "Agriculture EU" with a green label featuring the image of a leaf outlined by white dots.

The second thing you need to be aware of is the origin of the oil and how it is shipped to your destination. Make sure your importer or distributor deals with reputable growers and distillers and that the oils are temperature controlled and not shipped in barrels sitting in the hot tropical or desert sun. I know this is a lot to think about, but remember that these are essential oils you are going to put on your body; knowing as much as you can about them and how they are processed and shipped can make a huge difference in your health. Don't use any oil that is cheap or marginal on your precious body.

---

37 "What is Organic Agriculture?" www.usda.gov/wps/portal/usda/usdahome?contentidonly=true&contentid=organic-agriculture.html.

38 "US-EU Organic Equivalency Arrangement," www.usda-eu.org/trade-with-the-eu/trade-agreements/us-eu-organic-arrangement.

Labels

In the marketplace and online you will find essential oils claiming to be "Therapeutic," "Pure," "100 Percent Natural," "All Natural" "Made with Natural Products," "Made with Organic Products/Materials," "Pure and Natural," "Genuine," "100% Pure," "Holistic," "Home Grown," "(Name") Organics," "(Name) Naturals," "Scented with," and as many clever marketing word combinations as you can think of.

These terms mean nothing. "Organic" or "100 Percent Organic" and "Certified" are the words you are looking for. Check for the "Certified Organic" stamp, which should be printed on the label of an organic product. If the oils are from Europe, look for the verbiage "Agriculture EU" with a green label featuring a leaf outlined by white dots.

The FDA governs how aromatherapy products are categorized and how they can be labeled and sold to consumers. The FDA determines a product's intended use based on factors such as claims made in the labeling, on websites, and in advertising, as well as what consumers expect it to do. So we must look at how a product is marketed and not just a word or phrase taken out of context.

Is it a cosmetic?

If a product is intended only to cleanse the body or to make a person more attractive, it's a cosmetic. So, if a product such as a shower gel is intended only to cleanse the body, or a perfume or cologne is intended only to make a person smell good, it's a cosmetic.

Is it a drug?

If a product is intended for a therapeutic use such as treating or preventing disease, or to affect the structure or function of the body, it's a drug. For example, claims that a product will relieve colic, ease pain, relax muscles, treat depression or anxiety, or help you sleep are drug claims.

Under the law, drugs must meet requirements such as FDA approval for safety and effectiveness before they go on the market.

Is it both a cosmetic and a drug?

Some products are both cosmetics and drugs. For example, a baby lotion marketed with claims that it both moisturizes the baby's skin and relieves colic would be both a cosmetic and a drug. Such products must meet the requirements for both cosmetics and drugs.

If an essential oil or other fragrance is natural or organic, doesn't that mean it is safe?

Sometimes people think that if an essential oil or other ingredient comes from a plant, it must be safe. But many plants contain materials that are toxic, irritating, or likely to cause allergic reactions when applied to the skin.

For example, food grade cumin oil is safe in food, but when applied to the skin can cause blistering. Certain citrus oils used safely in food can also be harmful in cosmetics, particularly when applied to skin exposed to the sun.

Safety

Organic essential oils are the purest oils available. If we hold our essential oils in high regard and have respect for them, we will treat them as the special creations they are. Be sure to familiarize yourself thoroughly with the properties and uses of each essential oil you intend to use and make note of its cautions. Also check several sources for safety and precautions as some sensitivities can occur depending on a person's chemistry and reaction to oil extracts.

Never take essential oils internally! The only exception to this would be when the use of the oil is under the supervision of a certified aromatherapist. (There are a few suggestions for internal consumption in this book, but you will need to intake them only under proper supervision.) NAHA.org provides a list of qualified aromatherapists.

Never use essential oils undiluted on the skin. There are three oils that are commonly thought to be "safe" for using neat (undiluted) on your skin: lavender, tea tree, and chamomile essential oil. Forget that. All essential oils are condensed and strong. It is best to never use undiluted essential oils on your skin unless you are under the supervision of a certified Aromatherapist. Always perform a patch test on your skin before using oils as there are recorded instances of allergic reaction and sensitization even to the most innocuous oils. Essential oils should be diluted before application, even for a patch test.

Patch Test

Open the essential oil bottle. Dilute a drop or two in a carrier oil. (See the dilution charts beginning on page 50 for guidance.) Gently dip a toothpick or cotton swab into the mixture and extract a small drop of the diluted oil. Have a bottle of olive oil nearby. Apply a smidgen to your arm or leg and watch how your skin reacts. If there is a negative reaction *of any kind,* immediately cleanse the area with olive oil and wipe away the essential oil. Do not rinse with soap and water as this may aggravate the condition and spread the irritation.

Another method is to place the dab of diluted oil on the inside of your elbow and cover it with a bandage for twenty-four hours. When you remove the bandage the next day, if there is no reaction, then the essential oil is considered safe for you to use.[39] If you do discover a reaction (redness, swelling, soreness), there may be a couple of reasons for it: You could be allergic to the essential oil and its chemical components, or there are toxic materials, pesticides, or other impurities in the essential oil. You can further dilute the essential oil in a carrier oil and try the patch test again as dilution may also be the key, or you may find you are totally allergic to the oil and should avoid it entirely. Absolutely discontinue use of the essential oil if there is a negative reaction. In some rare cases the continued use of an essential oil can cause organ damage and hormonal imbalances.

More Cautions

When buying essential oils make sure that the bottles are sealed securely and have not been tampered with.

Always adhere to recommended safety standards and recommended dilution ratios. Never put essential oils directly into your eyes. Damage can occur to the cornea if oils are put directly into the eye. Be very careful when applying essential oils to the face and avoid the eye region altogether. There are many delicate tissues around the eyes.

If you are pregnant or nursing, consult a qualified Aromatherapist and your physician for the suitability and safety of specific oils. Many oils should not be used during pregnancy; some only need to be avoided for the first three to four months, others may be helpful during labor, but otherwise may pose a threat. The best idea is to seek professional

---

39 Aroma Web Essential Oil Skin Patch Test, www.aromaweb.com/articles/essential-oil-skin
-patch-test.asp.

help before using them. Refer to the paper written by the International Federation of Professional Aromatherapists on pregnancy in the resources section at the back of the book.

If you have a serious medical condition such as (but not limited to) asthma, high blood pressure, heart disease, kidney or liver disease, cancer, thrombosis, varicose veins, mental illness, or epilepsy, consult a qualified Aromatherapist for professional advice on recommended oils and dosages.

Essential oils are strong, even diluted, and can have an effect on medical conditions. If you are taking medications for a serious medical condition, there can be interactions with essential oils. Please consult a qualified Aromatherapist and your medical doctor before engaging in the use of essential oils.

One of my early teachers told our class that one drop of peppermint essential oil was the equivalent of twenty-eight cups of peppermint tea. When you start using essential oils, it is important that you know these are strong and potent essences not to be used without caution and proper dilution. It's just a matter of being safe and sane when using these amazing essential oils.

Taking care of yourself and being proactive with alternative therapies is a positive thing to do. But, if your symptoms persist or re-occur, or you are suffering from a severe or chronic medical condition or are presently taking prescription drugs, I recommend that you consult both a medical doctor and a qualified aromatherapy consultant before attempting to help yourself. The ideal is to find a practitioner as well as a doctor you can trust and who is prepared to work with you in exploring natural health alternatives.

Child Safety

Essential oils are strong. Using them with babies and children has rules, followed by common sense. Here are some guidelines for you to follow:

- Essential oils are powerful compounds and although they are natural extracts from various botanical material, they are highly concentrated, and should never be left where children or animals can get to them.

- Skin application and direct inhalations should be avoided for children under five years old.

- Do not use peppermint essential oil on children under five years old.

- Avoid ravensara on children under ten.

- Keep your essential oils in a safe childproof place. Keep them out of reach of tiny hands but also in a cool dark place that will help to prolong the life of your essential oils. I suggest a locking box that only adults can reach and access. Keep away from pets and animals, too.

- **Always use a weaker dilution on children:** Their bodies are smaller and their skin is more sensitive. When preparing a blend for a child, remember that you would halve the strength—where you would normally include a 2 percent dilution of essential oil to the carrier oil, you would prepare a 1 percent dilution for use on a child. **For example:** in adults you might use 5–6 drops of essential oil to 20 ml carrier oil, while on children you would only use 2–3 drops to 20 ml of carrier oil.

- If you are using a diffusion blend with children, do not leave them unattended with the diffuser, and only diffuse for one minute at a time with children under twelve years of age. Also be advised that animals are sensitive to diffused essential oils and make sure there is plenty of circulating air when you diffuse and keep the diffusion away from your pet's water bowls and sleeping area.

- For children under two, you can use hydrosols instead of essential oils. Hydrosols (floral waters, hydroflorates, flower waters, or distillates) are products obtained from steam distilling plant materials. Hydrosols are like essential oils but in a far less potent concentration.

Essential oils NOT to use on children or without the advice of a qualified Aroma-therapist:

Basil	Bay	Benzoin
Bergamot	Birch	Black pepper
Cassia	Cedarwood	Cinnamon
Citronella	Clove	Costus
Cumin	Elecampane	Eucalyptus
Fennel	Fir	Ginger
Helichrysum	Juniper	Lemon
Lemon verbena	Lemongrass	Melissa
Nutmeg	Oak moss	Orange
Oregano	Parsley seed	Peppermint
Pimento berry	Pine	Tagetes
Thyme (red)[40]		

Phototoxic Essential Oils

Some essential oils are phototoxic; you should not go out into the sunlight, use tanning beds, or subject yourself to ultraviolet rays for twelve to eighteen hours after use:

Angelica root	Bitter orange	Cumin
Dill	Grapefruit	Laurel leaf
Lemon	Lemon verbena	Lime
Mandarin	Orange	Rue
Tagetes	Tangerine	Yuzu[41]

The use of these essential oils in combination with exposure to the sun or UV rays can result in sunburn, blisters, edema (tissue swelling), or changes in the color of your skin.

---

40 "Safety," www.naha.org/explore-aromatherapy/safety.

41 Robert Tisserand and Rodney Young, *Essential Oil Safety: A Guide for Health Care Professionals* (London: Churchill Livingstone, 2013), 659.

Toxic Essential Oils

Below is a partial list of essential oils that are toxic, according to my collection of sources, the writings of Tisserand and Young in their *Guide for Health Care Professionals* and several other aromatherapy course instructors including the NAHA.org site. These should never be taken internally or topically by a consumer without the guidance and supervision of a certified Aromatherapist.

Ajowan	Arnica	Bitter Almond
Sweet Birch	Boldo Leaf	Calamus
Camphor	Cassia	Deertongue
Garlic	Horseradish	Jaborandi
Melilotus	Mugwort	Mustard
Onion	Rue	Sassafras
Savin	Tansy	Thuja
Wintergreen	Wormseed	Wormwood[42]

Pregnancy

Below is a list of essential oils to avoid if you are pregnant or breastfeeding.

Anise star	Aniseed	Basil
Birch, sweet	Camphor	Cinnamon
Cumin	Hyssop	Mugwort
Oregano	Parsley seed or leaf	Pennyroyal
Sage	Savory	Tansy
Tarragon	Thuja	Thyme
Wintergreen	Wormwood[43]	

---

42 "Safety," naha.org.

43 "Safety" www.naha.org/explore-aromatherapy/safety/#pregnancy and www.naha.org/assets /uploads/PregnancyGuidelines-Oct11.pdf.

What you need to know is that the essential oils with the highest number of phenols are the ones to avoid during pregnancy and breastfeeding. Refer to the paper written by the International Federation of Professional Aromatherapists on pregnancy in the sources section at the back of the book.

Pets and Animals

Many people want to use essential oils on their animals. There are many sites and books that recommend it. There are also many cases of animal death, adverse reaction, and illness from the improper or overly potent use of essential oils. Unfortunately, there is not enough research to support use of essential oils on animals except by a certified Aromatherapist who specializes in animal care. If you want to use essential oils on your animals, please consult a certified Aromatherapist who has a good track record in animal care.[44] See also Kelly Holland Azzaro's website on animal and pet care in the sources section in the back of the book.

Cats are extremely sensitive to essential oils and can sustain kidney and liver damage due to the properties in the essential oils. Dogs and horses are less sensitive, but can be negatively affected by certain oils. Fish, birds, small mammals, and rodents are on the no-no list for use.

Summary

If you've already purchased an essential oil, or a few, and they don't match the above criteria, don't worry, unless they are on the toxic list. They will not go to waste. They can be used and diffused in careful ways that will not directly impact you in a negative way. When you go shopping you'll know how to make the right and best choices for yourself.

What constitutes a great essential oil is the sum of many factors such as the seeds or cuttings used to start the plants, the growing methods, harvesting methods, distillation process, and after-care (post-distillation). The fewer pesticides, the better for you and your family. I recommend that you look for a certified organic label and care for your precious essential oils as you would anything near and dear to your heart and your body.

---

44   Kelly Holland Azzaro, "Animal Aromatherapy and Essential Oil Safety," www.naha.org/assets /uploads/Animal_Aromatherapy_Safety_NAHA.pdf.

Pay attention to the cautions, get to know the oils individually and if you have any questions whatsoever about safety, consult a qualified Aromatherapist and a medical doctor.

Organically grown essential oils are on the rise; more and more distilleries are becoming better experienced in the art and science of distilling quality essential oils. The good news is that as the demand for quality and organic essential oils grows, so will the increase in production and availability—and the cost may level out, too.

SIX

Blending Essential Oils

You're probably ready to purchase a few essential oils and try them out. You'll need some carrier oils to go with your essential oils because they are so highly concentrated. We have already discussed the potency of the essential oils and you'll want to make sure you use them safely by diluting them in carrier oils that are less potent. (Remember that one drop of peppermint essential oil is equal to twenty-eight cups of peppermint tea.) The whole purpose of being a healing artist and using your own palette of essential oils is in mixing and defining your colors. The carrier oils should also be organic and pure for safety and health reasons. Essential oils can be used individually, or as you will read in the "uses" section later in this chapter, blended with other essential oils.

There are companies who manufacture blends that claim to bring you harmony, peace, and relief of this or that condition or ailment. I recommend you blend your own because that gives you complete control of the quality of essential oil that goes into your blend. You alone determine what your specific needs are and only you can assess how you respond to the various and very different essential oils. Choose organic essential oils, use sterile conditions, and allow enough time to combine and rest the blend before diluting or using it.

Tips for Blending

1. I recommend that you use only organic essential oils and organic carrier oils. This protects you from toxins or rancidity that can occur in the manufacturing and shipping of these concentrated essential oils.

2. Try to limit your blend to three or four essential oils for your first session.

3. Take into consideration the purpose of the blend. What are you trying to accomplish? Is it a blend for a diffuser, an inhaler, for massage, or for direct application to clear up a condition? Are you working on the physical, emotional, or spiritual level? Is this to heal yourself or another? Intention is very important.

4. If you are working on a fragrance blend, you may want to add a top note with a middle and a base note for your first effort.* (You don't have to follow this formula, but it may be helpful to you in the beginning.)

5. Use 3x5" cards to keeps a record of how many drops you used per each essential oil and for what purpose, so you can duplicate the blend if you absolutely love it.

6. Remember a little goes a long way. One drop at a time. You can always add more.

7. I firmly believe in creating your own blends and not purchasing blends already pre-mixed. Essential oils should be pure, organic, and the blends should come for your own inner healing wisdom and intuition as you learn more and more about the oils.

*Please refer to the back of this chapter for more details about the "notes" of essential oils.

Dilution

Dilution is as much a necessity as it is an art.

Essential oils are concentrated and potent. Most of them are too concentrated to use directly on the skin.

Essential oils should always be diluted in carrier oils (see list below). Always!

The percentage of dilution depends on the results you are trying to achieve. Follow these seven tips when diluting essential oils:

1. A .25 percent dilution (1 drop per 4 tsp. of carrier oil)—for children between six months and six years. It is recommended that you only use essential oils on children under the proper supervision of an Aromatherapist. For children under five, you can use hydrosols instead. Hydrosols, also known as floral waters, hydroflorates, flower waters, or distillates are products obtained from steam distilling plant materials. Hydrosols are like essential oils but in a far less potent concentration.

2. A 1 percent dilution (1 drop per tsp. of carrier oil; 5–6 drops per oz.)—for children over age six, pregnant women, the elderly, or people with compromised immune systems, sensitive skin, or other serious health issues. This is also the dilution to use for massaging a large area of the body.

3. A 2 percent dilution (2 drops per tsp. of carrier oil; 10–12 drops per oz.)—ideal for most adults and in most situations. It is also the recommended dilution for daily skin application and care.

4. A 3 percent dilution (3 drops per tsp. of carrier oil; 15–18 drops per oz.)—best used short-term for a temporary health issue, such as a muscle injury or respiratory congestion. Up to 10 percent dilution is acceptable, depending on the health concern, the age of the person and the oils being used. Always consult a certified Aromatherapist for strong dilutions.

5. A 25 percent dilution (25 drops per tsp. of carrier oil; 125–150 drops per oz.)—for special occasions a dilution of this strength may be warranted. Examples are: severe pain, bad bruising, or a muscle cramp. Always consult a certified Aromatherapist for strong dilutions.

6. **Safety tip:** Use the lowest dilution of essential oils possible. A little goes a long way and you can often experience great results with a small amount.

We dilute our essential oils because we want to use them carefully and responsibly. We also want to avoid irritation, phototoxicity, fetotoxicity, hepotoxicity, carcinogenicity neurotoxicity and sensitization.[45]

Sensitization means that you can develop a sensitivity to a particular essential oil that, in the most dramatic circumstances, can cause anaphylactic shock, respiratory issues, or adverse skin reactions. This sensitization can be permanent and cause a reaction to surface when you are near the essential oil. It is advisable to dilute every essential oil to prevent sensitization. Below is a chart you can use for diluting essential oils with carrier oils.

E.O.	C.O.	Dilution %
1 drop	in 1 tsp. (5ml)	= 1.0%
2 drops	in 1 tsp. (5ml)	= 2.0%
3 drops	in 1 tsp. (5ml)	= 3.0%
10 drops	in 1 tsp. (5ml)	= 10%
25 drops	in 1 tsp. (5ml)	= 25%
1 drop	in 2 tsp. (10ml)	= .05%
2 drops	in 2 tsp. (10ml)	= 1.0%
4 drops	in 2 tsp. (10ml	= 2.0%
6 drops	in 2 tsp. (10ml)	= 3.0%
20 drops	in 2 tsp. (10ml)	= 10%
50 drops	in 2 tsp. (10ml)	= 25%
3 drops	in ½ oz. (15ml)	= 1.0%
6 drops	in ½ oz. (15ml)	= 2.0%
9 drops	in ½ oz. (15ml)	= 3.0%
30 drops	in ½ oz. (15ml)	= 10%
75 drops	in ½ oz. (15ml)	= 25%

45   Robert Tisserand, learningabouteos.com.

E.O.	C.O.	Dilution %
3 drops	in 1 oz. (30ml)	= .05%
6 drops	in 1 oz. (30ml)	= 1.0%
12 drops	in 1 oz. (30ml)	= 2.0%
18 drops	in 1 oz. (30ml)	= 3.0%
60 drops	in 1 oz. (30ml)	= 10%
150 drops	in 1 oz. (30ml)	= 25%

Carrier Oils

- Jojoba oil, *Simmondsia chinensis*
- Sweet almond oil, *Prunus dulcis*
- Avocado oil, *Persea americana*
- Apricot kernel oil, *Prunus armeniaca*
- Carrot seed oil, *Daucus carota*
- Grapeseed oil, *Vitis vinifera*
- Virgin, cold pressed olive oil, *Olea europaea*
- Pomegranate oil, *Punica granatum*
- Fractionated coconut oil, *Cocos nucifera*
- Safflower oil, *Carthamus tinctorius*
- Sesame oil, *Sesamum indicum*
- Sunflower oil, *Helianthus annuus*
- Evening primrose oil, *Oenothera biennis*
- Borage seed oil, *Borago officinalis*
- Wheat germ oil, *Triticum vulgare*

I found that I most liked working with the top five carrier oils on the above list. Please experiment with your own carrier oils and find the one or two you enjoy the most. Be sure to find pure and organic carrier oils, just like the essential oils you buy.

There is a lot of advice available on the Internet about which oils to blend together and how to blend them according to the "notes" the essential oil possesses.

There are some recipes you can follow but let's begin by looking at the list of the essential oils and their categories first.

These classifications originated from George William Septimus Piesse in his book *The Art of Perfumery*. He also created the *odaphone*, a scent scale used to rank the odor of perfumes.

According to this scale, there are three note categories an essential oil can fall into: top, middle, or base. You may not care about combining essential oils for the sole purpose of blending for the perfume effect, but a fragrant combination works wonders for healing on every level.

Top Notes

Essential oils that are classified as top notes normally evaporate very fast. They are fast-acting and usually give the "first impression" of the blend you are making.

Basil	Bergamot	Clary sage
Eucalyptus	Grapefruit	Lemon
Lemongrass	Lime	Mandarin
Neroli	Orange	Peppermint
Petitgrain	Ravensara	Sage
Spearmint	Tagetes	Tangerine
Tea tree	Thyme	Verbena

Middle Notes

These oils give body to the blend and are balancers. The middle notes may not be immediately evident and may take a few minutes to be recognized.

They are usually warm and soft smelling.

Bay	Black pepper	Cardamom
Chamomile	Cypress	Fennel
Geranium	Juniper	Lavender
Marjoram	Melissa	Myrtle
Nutmeg	Palma rosa	Pine
Rosemary	Spikenard	Yarrow

Base Notes

They are normally heavy oils whose fragrances are quite evident and forward, but they also can evolve slowly and are potent for a longer time and slow the evaporation of the other oils. They are heady, intense, and can be costly.

Balsam peru	Cassia	Cedarwood
Cinnamon	Clove	Frankincense
Ginger	Jasmine	Myrrh
Patchouli	Rose	Sandalwood
Valerian	Vanilla	Vetiver
Ylang-ylang		

Remember to add only a drop of the strongly fragranced essential oil at a time to prevent it from overpowering your entire blend. Blending not only relies on the notes, but also on the purpose, measurement, and relationship of one oil to another. This is why your blending experimentations should be done with patience and a playful spirit.

Ways to Use the Blends

You can use the blends you create with essential oils in many ways.

1. **Diffusers:** The aromas of the essential oils are distributed throughout the room/house to provide emotional relief as well as therapeutic assistance like purification and disinfecting according to the properties of each essential oil. (Avoid using diffusers that require heat as this

method may harm the delicate essential oils.) There is a difference between a humidifier and a diffuser. You'll want to research diffusers that use water and essential oils and ones that use just essential oils. Read the manufacturer's recommendations for use and follow the guidelines.

2. **Inhalers:** These are personal and portable mini diffusers of essential oils you create to order for help with respiration, cold symptoms, allergies, stopping smoking, losing weight, controlling seasickness, uplifting a mood, or as a source of energy and stimulation.

3. **Baths:** mix essential oils with Epsom salts, another carrier oil, or even a little powdered, almond, or coconut milk to disperse in a bath for soothing, calming, and therapeutic benefits.

4. **Compresses:** Dilute essential oils in a carrier oil in warm or cool water. Submerge a washcloth and then wring out excess water. Apply compress to the area you want to assist, relieve, cool, or reduce pain.

5. **Massage:** Use 15 drops of your favorite essential oil(s) to 1 oz. of carrier oil. Massage over affected area of your body. For intense repair, you can use 30 drops to 1 oz. of carrier oil.

6. **Steam inhalation:** After you have boiled some water and turned off the stove, pour the hot water into a basin, add selected essential oils into the hot water, cover your head with a towel, close your eyes and, without burning yourself or your tender skin, inhale the steam for 5–10 minutes. This method is used for clearing the sinuses, reducing coughs, clearing congestions, and sore throats.

7. **Face and body creams:** You can prepare your own cosmetics and body creams using ingredients such as cocoa butter, shea butter, bees wax, and essential oils. The creams can be effective for scars, dry skin, wrinkles, and the suppleness of skin. There are recipes in chapter fourteen to help you get started in the process of infusing your entire

life with life-affirming essential oils. Always dilute and keep away from eye area. This is only the beginning. Your own creativity will take your life to a whole new level.

There is one more thing you should know:

Proper Disposal

Essential oils should not be disposed of in kitchen sinks, drains, or into any other receptacle that comes into contact with bodies of water, water supplies, pipelines, vegetation, or animals.

Placing a few drops of essential oil down your drain to freshen bad drain odors is okay, but only use a drop or two at a time. If your essential oil has outlived its shelf life apply a drop or two on dryer sheets, shelf liners (check the stain factor), in your trash container (inside and out), or even as a drain refresher, but only one or two drops at a time. Label them "old" or "past date" and gradually use the essential oils up on tasks like these.

Generally essential oils don't go bad, but some have longer lives than others. If your oil has been mixed with a synthetic oil or a carrier oil, it could shorten its life. I don't recommend using essential oils that are mixed or diluted with synthetic oils. You'll know if your oil has passed its mark if it smells off.

In general terms, my experience averages about nine to fourteen months with a citrus oil, nine to twenty months with carrier oils, and up to three years with other essential oils. The key to longevity is storing them in a cool, dark place with tightened caps. Heat, light, and air are the worst hazards of degradation for delicate essential oils.

Remember that essential oils are flammable and can be toxic to animals and creatures. Use them carefully and responsibly. Once you select and purchase an essential oil, you are in charge. Make sure you abide by the safety precautions, do patch tests for skin irritation, and keep yourself and your family safe from accidental ingestion.

PART TWO

The Healing Palette of 50 Essential Oils

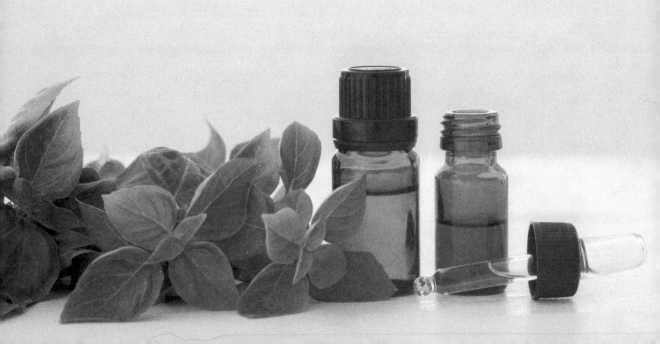

SEVEN

The Primary Palette of Essential Oils 1–12

We get to know people better when we ask questions about where they were born, what their family was like, how they were raised, and what their gifts and talents are. Essential oils are much the same. The more we know about their origin, their history, and show interest in their specific healing qualities, the more we will appreciate and understand them.

The beauty of essential oils is that there is no limit to the wealth of your own creations. You can use essential oils for yourself, your children, your friends, your cosmetics, your remedial needs and more. The more you experiment with essential oils, the more you will value them and the more they will do for you. Here are my choices for the first twelve that would be good to begin using for your primary palette as a healing artist approaching your first masterpiece.

1: Lavender

If you only could have one essential oil, lavender (*Lavandula angustifolia*), the most versatile of all essential oils and one of the most gentle, would be my choice. Most commonly known for its relaxing effects on the body and mind, lavender essential oil has been highly revered for healing the mind, body, and soul.

Its name originates from:

Latin: *Nardus/Lavandula vera*	**French:** *Lavande*
Spanish: *Alhucema/lavanda*	**English:** *Elf leaf/nard/lavender*
Gender: *Masculine*	**Ruling Planet:** *Mercury*
Element: *Air*	

Property Description

Antimicrobial, antibacterial, antifungal, antitumoral, anticonvulsant, relaxant, anti-inflammatory, nervine

Benefits

Calming, relaxing, balancing, improves mental acuity

Possessing antibacterial and antimicrobial properties, lavender essential oil can soothe cuts and burns as well as treat fungal infections due to its powerful antiseptic properties. These same properties do wonders for the hair and scalp. It even works (when used with other essential oils) as a natural bug repellant. Lavender essential oil is also a wonderful remedy for insomnia, motion sickness, stress, anxiety, fatigue, and headaches.

Research finds that exposing yourself to the scent of lavender reduces postoperative pain, childbirth pain, and menstrual cramps.

> The aroma of lavender increases alpha waves, or *slow waves*, in the back of the head, which has a relaxing effect. By making people more relaxed, it makes people less anxious, which is significant because anxiety increases pain.[46]

Background

Ancient records regarding the lavender plant have been found in Greece, where the flower took the name of its birthplace from the Syrian city of Naarda and was originally

---

46   Marla Paul, "Common Scents," articles.chicagotribune.com/1995–11–19/features/9511190164
_1_smell-taste-treatment-neurological-director-common-scents.

called referred to as *nardus*.[47] The name "lavender" itself is a derivative of the Latin word *lavare*, meaning "to wash." It was used by the Romans as a perfume for their baths and was also added to their washing agents because it perfumed their clothes with its pleasant and soothing aroma.

The floral fragrance has been used by many cultures for centuries because it has therapeutically calming, relaxing, and balancing properties that register physically and emotionally. Historically, it has many uses and success stories. Lavender has been used as a perfume, in cooking, as an aid for depression, as an immune system builder, and for anxiety and fatigue relief. It is also highly famous for its skin-healing properties.

COMMON USES FOR LAVENDER ESSENTIAL OIL

- Soothe minor skin burns with 2 to 3 drops of diluted lavender essential oil.

- Rub lavender essential oil lip balm on sunburned, dry, or chapped skin and lips to moisturize and to minimize scar tissue.

- A single drop diluted on a minor cut can also kill bacteria while helping to stop the bleeding and heal the wound.

- A single drop diluted will reduce the itching of a bee sting or a cold sore.

- Mix several drops of lavender essential oil with a pure carrier oil and use topically for skin conditions like eczema and dermatitis.

- Diffuse a few drops of lavender essential oil to minimize the effects of hay fever, pollen, seasonal change, and air quality discomforts.

- To chase off and repel bugs: mix 15 drops of lavender essential oil and 5 drops of eucalyptus essential oil in 2 T of carrier oil and rub on your skin.

- To stop a nosebleed, place a drop of diluted lavender essential oil on a soft tissue and cover a small chip of ice. Push the tissue covered ice chip up and under the middle of the top lip until it almost touches the base

---

47 "Lavender," www.herbs-info.com/lavender.html.

of your nose and hold it as long as comfortable or until the bleeding stops. Be careful not to freeze your lip or gum.[48]

- Alleviate the symptoms of motion sickness by placing a drop of diluted lavender essential oil behind your ears or around your navel.

- Apply a few drops of diluted lavender essential oil to your hands and rub on a child's pillow to assist him/her with sleep. (Child should be over six months old).

- Diffuse lavender essential oil to set the mood for pleasant social gatherings.

- Diffuse or inhale lavender essential oil at the end of the day to release tension and refresh your mind, body, and spirit.

- Rub 2–3 drops of diluted lavender essential oil in your cupped palms, then inhale the scent to establish calm, invoke sleep, or even relieve hay fever.

- Rub diluted mixture on your feet, temples, wrists, or anywhere to bring about an immediate calming effect, or to minimize dandruff massage into your scalp.

- Use diluted lavender essential oil in crowded areas like planes or subways to create your personal oasis and in hotel rooms to aid tranquility and help your body adapt to a strange location.

- Create more restful sleep by inhaling a few drops of diluted lavender essential oil rubbed into the palms of your hands and then smoothed onto your pillow to help you sleep.

- Place a few drops of lavender essential oil on a wet cloth or add to a dryer sheet to deodorize and freshen your laundry.

- Repel moths and insects by adding a few drops of lavender essential oil to cotton balls and place them in closets and drawers.

---

48   Karen Zuckerman, "How Do Essential Oils Work?," www.karenzuckerman.com/main .htm#topic44.

- Scent your linen drawer in the same way as above using a saturated cotton ball of lavender essential oil.

- Make sachets out of lavender essential oil doused cotton balls.

Cautions

Lavender essential oil is one of the safest essential oils you can use. A standard caution is not to use for infants under the age of six months. Some physicians caution to not use it two weeks prior to surgery. And there have been some side effects when used on teens.

Blends Well With

Bergamot, black pepper, cedarwood, Roman chamomile, clary sage, clove bud, eucalyptus, geranium, grapefruit, lemon, lemongrass, marjoram, patchouli, peppermint, ravensara, rose, rosemary, tea tree, thyme, and vetiver essential oils.

Supernatural Uses

In occult and magical practice, lavender essential oil is used to attract love, incite prophetic dreams, open the third eye, stimulate the seventh chakra, and encourage the appearance of spirits. Lavender has historically been used as a gift offering to various deities and as a form of incense for cleansing and consecration.

- For wishes to come true, place drops of lavender essential oil on your pillow as you bring the wish to mind. (Test for oil staining.)

- Infuse clothing with lavender essential oil to attract love.

- Drop some lavender essential oil on stationery to write love notes.

- Wear lavender essential oil on clothing to promote long life.

2: Tea Tree

Tea tree (*Melaleuca alternifolia*) was named by a group of eighteenth-century sailors who made a pot of tea from the leaves of a tree they found when they came ashore on the south coast of Australia. It smelled like nutmeg to them so they called it "tea tree." Tea tree essential oil is derived from the leaves of the tea tree.[49]

---

49 "Tea Tree," www.cloverleaffarmherbs.com/tea-tree/.

Its name originates from:

Latin: *Melaleuca alternifolia*	**French:** *arbre à thé*
Spanish: *aceite del árbol del té*	**English:** *Tea tree oil*
Gender: *Feminine*	**Ruling Planet:** *Jupiter*
Element: *Fire*	

Property Description

Bactericide, antiviral, cicatrisant, antifungal, antiseptic, expectorant, stimulant, antimicrobial.

Benefits

Tea tree essential oil is known to be cleansing, purifying, and uplifting. It is used externally for a number of conditions ranging from acne to athlete's foot, nail fungus, infections and wounds; as a lice abatement, for oral candidiasis (thrush), cold sores, dandruff, and as a relief for skin lesions.

Tea tree is a very safe essential oil having a strong, camphorous, balsamic, and pungent odor emanating from the plant leaves. It has potent and effective antibacterial, antifungal, and antiviral properties. Therefore it is a *must* in a home healing cabinet. Tea tree essential oil is best used externally unless you are working with a trained Aromatherapist.

Background

This tree is native to Australia, specifically Queensland and New South Wales, and its oil has been known and used among the natives as a universal medicinal remedy since ancient times. Aborigines in the area ground up the leaves to make a salve for skin wounds. The leaves are also used as a tea to help cure respiratory ailments. Travelers to Australia spread the word about the healing properties of the plant in the 1920s and suddenly the world wanted to know more. In the past ninety years numerous studies have tested tea tree oil's effects on skin ailments, infections, rashes and have concluded that it is a potentially viable treatment for certain conditions.[50]

---

50 "Tea Tree Oil," www.webmd.com/vitamins-supplements/ingredientmono-113–tea%20 tree%20oil.aspx?activeingredientid=113&activeingredientname=tea%20tree%20oil.

The characterization of this oil as a cure-all is not hyperbole. Tea tree oil can be used for a host of infections and diseases. The healing and disinfectant properties make it a wonder remedy that can boost immunity. However, it is not meant to be ingested because, used internally, it can turn to poison. Use topically only.[51]

Tea tree oil is twelve times stronger than phenol, a common disinfectant used in hospitals.[52]

COMMON USES FOR TEA TREE ESSENTIAL OIL

- Apply 2–3 drops of diluted tea tree essential oil to soothe minor burns. It will also help prevent scars from forming.

- A drop or 2 of diluted tea tree essential oil applied to the face as a bacterial wash will help break-outs and blemished skin. One dab on acne can reduce redness and swelling.

- For a refreshing massage dilute 10 drops of tea tree essential oil in 1 oz. of carrier oil and massage over the body for tension and stress relief.

- Added to your mouthwash, a few drops of tea tree essential oil can help alleviate mouth infection or inflamed gums. (Avoid swallowing.)

- Eczema and dermatitis respond well to a mix of several drops of tea tree essential oil with a pure carrier oil and applied to the affected area.*

- Add tea tree essential oil to bath water to treat bronchial congestion, hacking cough, and pulmonary inflammation. Dilute with 1 T Epsom salts.

- Congestion can also be alleviated by rubbing a drop of diluted tea tree essential oil between your palms and inhaling deeply to help alleviate your symptoms.

---

51   K. A. Hammer, C. Carson, T. Riley, J. Nielsen, "A Review of the Toxicity of *Melaleuca alternifolia* (Tea Tree) Oil," journals.elsevier.com/food-and-chemical-toxicology.

52   "Interesting Facts about Tee Tree Oil," www.defensesoap.com/tea-tree-oil-facts-links-menu-dont-publish-269.html.

- Diluted tea tree essential oil is effective for persistent coughs when used in inhalers and diffusers. Diffuse a few drops of tea tree essential oil to ease chest congestion or add 4 drops of tea tree essential oil to an open pan of boiling water, cover your head with a towel, close your eyes, and inhale the steam to alleviate congestion, colds, and coughs. (Don't bend too close to the steaming pan to avoid burns.)

- Head lice can be destroyed by adding a small amount of tea tree essential oil to shampoo.

- Freshen up fabrics using a spray bottle mixed with 2 C of water and 2 T of tea tree essential oil. Test the fabric for staining, then spray the stale-smelling area and let it rest for a few days. Most of the musty scent and the pungent tea tree essential oil smell will dissipate.

- An all-purpose cleaner can be created by adding 2 tsp. of tea tree essential oil to 2 C of water in a clean spray bottle. Shake well before using each time. This same mixture will also control mold growth.

- For sanitized and germ-free dishes and glasses, add a few drops of tea tree essential oil to dishwasher dispenser, then fill with a biodegradable dishwashing soap.

- Adding a few drops of tea tree essential oil to your laundry leaves your clothes smelling cleaner and helps to keep the storage bugs away.

- **To repel insects:** add 10 to 20 drops of tea tree essential oil to 2 T carrier oil and 1 T aloe vera gel. Reapply every 2 to 4 hours.

- Use a tiny drop of diluted tea tree essential oil neat on blisters or insect bites.

Cautions

Diluted tea tree essential oil is probably safe for most people when applied to the skin, but it can cause skin irritation and swelling. When using for acne, it can sometimes cause skin dryness, itching, stinging, burning, and redness.

Do a patch test on your skin to determine sensitivity. Be sure to keep it away from your eyes when applying to the face. You may experience redness and irritation if you use too close to the delicate eye tissue. Keep away from the eyes.

*There have been some cases of aggravation reported for cases of eczema. Do yourself the favor of a patch test before experimenting willy-nilly.

Blends Well With
Cinnamon, clary sage, clove bud, geranium, lavender, lemon, myrrh, rosemary, marjoram, and thyme essential oils.

Supernatural Uses
In occult and magical practice, tea tree essential oil is used to enhance strength; to cleanse, protect, and purify; and to open and focus the channels of the mind for more clarity. It is also used for opening up the upper chakras.

- When you need extra strength, place a drop of tea tree essential oil on a 1" piece of cloth to carry with you in situations where you could use some extra courage.

- Inhale 2 drops of tea tree essential oil rubbed on the palms of your hands to open upper chakras and for increasing mental clarity.

- Cleanse away all negative energies by adding a drop of tea tree essential oil to a cotton ball and inhaling the aroma three times.

3: Rosemary

Rosemary (*Rosmarinus officinalis*) is very popular in countries and cultures around the Mediterranean. Regional dishes are cooked with rosemary oil and garnished with freshly plucked rosemary leaves. Rosemary essential oil is mostly extracted from the leaves. The stems and branches of the plant can be used in cooking, allowing the flavor and smoke from the wood to permeate the food. The rosemary bush is part of the mint family, which includes basil, lavender, myrtle, and sage.

Its name originates from:

Latin: *Rosmarinus officinalis*	**French:** *Romarin*
Spanish: *Romero*	**English:** *Rosemary, compass weed, dew of the sea, elf leaf, guardrobe, incensier, sea dew*
Gender: *Masculine*	
Element: *Fire*	
	Ruling Planet: *Sun*

Propert Description

Astringent, analgesic, carmitive, detox, diuretic, memory enhancer, antirheumatic, tonic, stimulant.

Benefits

Restorative, purifying, protective, reviving, refreshing. Encourages relief from aching muscles, arthritis, dull skin, exhaustion, gout, dandruff, hair and scalp thinning, neuralgia, poor circulation, acne, and impaired memory, and aids weight loss.

Background

The Romans used rosemary in religious ceremonies and for blessings at weddings. Rosemary was an all-around herb, given special importance and used in food preparation, cosmetic care, and for medicinal purposes. The Romans weren't the first to capture its fragrance. The ancient Egyptians cornered its qualities long before then for use as fragrant incense. In Shakespeare's *Hamlet*, Ophelia says:

> There's rosemary, that's for remembrance. Pray you, love, remember.
> (Act IV, scene 5)[53]

The name "rosemary" derives from the Latin for dew (*ros*) and sea (*marinus*), rendering it "*dew of the sea.*" The plant is also sometimes called *anthos* from the ancient Greek word meaning *flower*. According to legend, the goddess Aphrodite had rosemary wrapped around her body when she rose up from the sea. It is believed that when the

---

53   *Hamlet* at nfs.sparknotes.com/hamlet/page_248.html.

Virgin Mary was resting, she spread her blue cloak over a white-blossomed rosemary bush for safe keeping, and the flowers miraculously turned a matching blue. The shrub then became known as the "Rose of Mary."[54]

Paracelsus, a renowned German-Swiss physician and botanist, made significant contributions to the understanding of herbal medicine during the sixteenth century. Paracelsus valued rosemary essential oil because of its ability to strengthen the entire body. He used it extensively because he found that rosemary essential oil had the ability to heal delicate organs such as the liver, brain, and heart.[55]

And in Hungary, Queen Isabella also contributed to rosemary's reputation as a rejuvenating tonic. She created what is known as Royal Hungarian Water, which is made by distilling rosemary, lavender, rose petals, orange flower, and lemon balm.[56]

A study conducted by the Herbal Medicine Department of the Tai Sophia Institute in 2012 tested the effect of rosemary leaf powder on people over the age of seventy-five. It found that the amount of the dosage taken played a pivotal role in how the participants' memory functioned.[57]

When selecting your rosemary essential oil, there is one more thing to make note of: chemotype. Rosemary has six. We will address the three major ones. Each chemotype brings with it different healing properties and potential sensitivities. The chemotype is abbreviated as "ct."

1. *Rosmarinus officinalis ct. camphor* is high in ketones and works best for muscle aches and pains, and massage relief. It addresses rheumatism discomfort and has diuretic and circulatory benefits.

2. *Rosmarinus officinalis ct. 1,8–cineole* is high in oxides. It is antiviral, antifungal, antibacterial, anti-inflammatory, cephalic, cardiotonic,

---

54 "Rosemary is for Remembrance," www.anzacday.org.au/education/tff/rosemary.html.

55 "Essential Oils," www.goldennaturals.com/blogs/essentialoils.

56 "Materia Aromatica Rosemary," materiaaromatica.com/Default.aspx?go=Article &ArticleID=213.

57 "Scientists Finding Sniffing Rosemary Can Increase Memory by 75%," www .healthyandnaturalworld.com/scientists-find-sniffing-rosemary-can-increase-memory/.

neurotonic, antirheumatic, anticatarrhal, carminative, expectorant, digestive stimulant, and hepatic stimulant. It is the better choice for alleviating respiratory and mucous issues. Added to shampoo, it can restore vitality to dull hair and works as a blood stimulator when massaged into the head.

3. *Rosmarinus officinalis ct. verbenone* is best used on the skin because it has ketones and monoterpenes, which inhibit the accumulation of toxins. It has antispasmodic benefits and is anti catarrhal, expectorant, cicatrisant, antibacterial, antidepressive, anti-infectious, antirheumatic, calmative, and cardiotonic. It can also be used successfully for respiratory issues.

If that sounds all too confusing, just remember to focus on what you want to solve and then back into your choice by checking out what each chemotype can do to suit your needs.

Common uses for Rosemary Essential Oil

- Rub several drops of diluted rosemary (ct. 1,8–cineole) essential oil into the scalp to help eliminate dandruff after washing your hair.

- **If you are looking to improve your memory:** mix together 3 drops of rosemary (ct. 1,8–cineole) essential oil with 1 tsp. of pure grade coconut oil, and rub on upper neck or diffuse alone (minus the coconut oil) for one hour a day.

- **If your hair is thinning:** use rosemary (ct. 1,8–cineole) essential oil as a hair thickener. Put 5 drops of diluted rosemary (ct. 1,8–cineole) essential oil on scalp and massage in after each shower.

- **To reduce joint and muscle pain:** mix 2 drops of rosemary (ct. camphor or ct. verbenone) essential oil, 2 drops of peppermint essential oil, and 1 T of carrier oil and rub on sore muscles and painful joints.

- Used externally, rosemary (ct. camphor or ct. verbenone) essential oil can help soothe the stomach and relieve pain from indigestion, menstrual cramps, or other difficulties. Dilute in a carrier oil and rub onto torso in a clockwise motion.

- **To assist gallbladder function:** mix together 3 drops of rosemary (ct. 1,8–cineole) essential oil with ¼ tsp. of carrier oil and massage over gallbladder area twice daily clockwise.

- **To relieve neuropathy and neuralgia discomfort:** add 2 drops of rosemary (ct. 1,8–cineole) essential oil, to 3 drops of helichrysum essential oil, 3 drops of cypress essential oil, and 1 tsp. of a carrier oil and rub on area of neuropathy.

- **For improved prostate health:** mix 2 drops of rosemary (ct. verbenone) essential oil with 1 T of carrier oil and rub underneath testicles.

- Rub rosemary essential oil (ct. verbenone) on your feet, temples, wrists, or anywhere to bring about an immediate calming effect in your whole body. Dilute in a carrier oil.

- Add a few drops of rosemary essential oil to a dryer sheet to deodorize and freshen your laundry. A wet cloth works just as well.

- Diffusing a few drops of rosemary essential oil (ct. verbenone or ct. 1,8–cineole) aids circulation, liver function, and as a stimulant, encourages weight loss.[58]

- **For super-effective weight loss:** make an inhaler and use it five times a day to discourage appetite. I suggest rosemary, black pepper, and pink grapefruit to help quell appetite. (Follow inhaler instructions in chapter fourteen.)

---

58   Sharon Lovett, "Essential Oils That Your Liver will Love," www.baseformula.com /blog/2012/01/essential-oils-that-your-liver-will-love/.

Cautions

Rosemary essential oil should not be used by pregnant women. According to the safety notes on AromaWeb, authors Tisserand and Young warn that:

> "Rosemary oil is potentially neurotoxic, depending on the level of camphor present in the oil."

They also warn not to use on or near the face of infants and children.[59] For this reason the second two versions are the safest to use: ct. verbenone or ct. 1,8–cineole.

Blends Well With

Frankincense, lavender, clary sage, cedarwood, basil, thyme, lemongrass, geranium, Roman chamomile, and peppermint essential oils.

Supernatural Uses

Used to bring protection, love, lust, enhanced mental powers, exorcism of evil spirits, purification, healing, sleep, and as an agent for youth.

- Use a few drops of rosemary essential oil in hotel rooms to increase safety and help your body adapt to a strange location.

- A drop of rosemary essential oil on a cloth under your pillow will help chase nightmares away.

- If you'd like an answer to a question, burn a drop of rosemary essential oil on a charcoal brick, gently inhale a bit of the smoke, and the answer will come to you.

- Diffuse a few drops of rosemary essential oil to increase mental clarity and raise feelings of safety and protection.

- Keep a cotton ball with two drops of rosemary essential oil handy when you are concentrating hard and need to break away to sniff every hour for refreshment and clarity.

---

59   "Rosemary Essential Oil," www.aromaweb.com/essential-oils/rosemary-oil.asp.

4: Lemon

The earliest lemons originated in China and were transported on ships by ancient explorers and merchants returning from east Asia with their goods and spices destined for Italy and the Mediterranean.

Its name originates from:

Latin: *Citrus limonum*	**French:** *Citron*
Spanish: *Limon*	**English:** *Lemon, ulamula*
Gender: *Feminine*	**Ruling Planet:** *Moon*
Element: *Water*	

Property Description

Astringent, antiseptic, bactericide, detoxifier, depurative, hypotensive, antimicrobial, antibacterial, autoimmune support, antifungal.

Benefits

Stimulating, calming, carminative, prevents infection, detoxifying, sleep inducing, digestive, disperses cellulite, wrinkle wrangler, and refreshing. Helps with varicose veins, parasites, and anxiety, as well as anxiety-induced headaches, hypertension, circulation problems, and obesity.

Background

A fruit that closely resembles a lemon is depicted in some of the most treasured Pompeian antique mosaics.[60] Botanists argue that lemons weren't well known in Europe until the Crusades. The earliest record of the lemon in the New World arrived with Christopher Columbus in 1492.[61] These seafaring adventurers sailed the seven seas and used fresh lemons to prevent scurvy. By the sixteenth century, the lemon had become commonplace.

---

60   "Lemon Oil," www.auracacia.com/auracacia/aclearn/eo_lemon.html.

61   Maureen Katemopoulous, "The History of Lemon Trees," www.gardenguides.com/126175 –history-lemon-trees.html.

Extremely sensitive to cold temperatures and high humidity, lemons are agriculturally best suited to the milder climates of southern California, Florida, and the Mediterranean region, where they now grow in abundant, fragrant orchards.

Lemons are extensively used in cooking and healing. In her 1931 book on herbal medicine, Maude Grieve wrote: "The lemon is the most valuable of all fruit for preserving health." Lemons are invigorating, cleansing, uplifting and inspiring. We can use lemon essential oil for a variety of purposes.

COMMON USES FOR LEMON ESSENTIAL OIL

- Sore throat pain and swelling can be reduced by adding a drop of organic lemon essential oil to your hot tea, or in warm water combined with honey. Be sure you do this under the supervision of a qualified Aromatherapist.

- **To ease coughs, colds, and general congestion:** a few drops of diluted lemon essential oil rubbed on your chest and/or throat will help relieve congestion. Diffuse a few drops of lemon essential oil to alleviate any other respiratory complaints.

- **For treating allergies and hay fever:** use well-diluted lemon essential oil (1 drop) behind the ear or under the nose two to three times a day to help fight seasonal allergies. (**Note:** stay out of the sunlight if you apply topically.) Alternatively, you can apply diluted lemon essential oil to the bottoms of your feet using a roller ball applicator. (Make sure you patch test for skin sensitivity.)

- Keep your toothbrush germ-free by using 1 drop of lemon essential oil on your toothbrush and twirling it in a bit of water to sanitize. Rinse well.

- 4 drops of lemon essential oil added to 4 oz. of warm water becomes a cleansing gargle for bad breath. It also is an effective mouthwash for mouth sores. Do not swallow.

- **To treat acne:** apply three drops of diluted lemon essential oil to a cotton ball and cleanse the affected area, repeating up to three times a day. Be careful of sun exposure after use on face.

- **To get windows that shine without streaks:** mix 50 percent water with 50 percent vinegar and add 10 to 20 drops lemon essential oil into a spray bottle. Shake well before using, spray, and wipe clean with paper towels. (You may find that it takes a skootch more time to dry the surface than with commercial cleaners, but you have the advantage of a chemical- and alcohol-free cleaner.)

- **For a general disinfectant around the house:** mix 3 drops lemon essential oil into 2 oz. of water and shake vigorously before wiping down wooden furniture and kitchen chopping blocks. Use a stronger mixture as a kitchen board sanitizer.

- **For a pick-me-up:** moisten a cloth with five drops of lemon essential oil and 5 drops of water. Hold cloth directly underneath your nose and breathe in the scent for at least 2 to 3 minutes.

- **For effective stress relief:** add 10 to 15 drops of lemon essential oil to your bath water and soak for at least 15 minutes. Adding a few drops of lavender essential oil increases stress relief. Avoid sun exposure after your bath.

- **For treating minor wounds:** place 5 drops of lemon essential oil in a bowl of 3 oz. of clean, warm water. Dip a sterilized cloth in the mixture and gently wipe the wound until it is clean.

- **Use to remove calluses, corns, and warts:** apply a drop of diluted lemon essential oil twice a day until they disappear.[62]

---

62 Adrienne Percy, "How to Cure a Plantar Wart Naturally," nourishedroots.ca/how-to-cure-a-plantar-wart-naturally.

- **To eradicate nail fungus:** apply 2 to 3 drops of diluted lemon essential oil to the nail in question several times a day. **Note:** Have patience. It may take a few weeks or even months for the fungus to fully clear up.

- **For a brighter skin and complexion:** add a drop or 2 of lemon essential oil to your nighttime moisturizer. It's very important that you do not do this in the morning since lemon oil (and most citrus oils) increase your sensitivity to the sun.

- **For a clearer mind:** diffuse a few drops of lemon essential oil in your office or study space to enhance mental clarity and concentration.

- Add a few drops of lemon essential oil plus 2 tsp. baking soda to your toilet to clean and sanitize the bowl.

- Rub a few drops of lemon essential oil on cutting boards and surfaces, knife handles, and other kitchen areas to sanitize them.

- Rid yourself of more kitchen germs by soaking kitchen cloths and rags for 12 hours in a bowl of water containing 2 to 3 drops of lemon essential oil.

- Add 8 drops to a diffuser and let the lemon essential oil clean and freshen the air. This also helps decongest lungs in cold and flu season.

- **Improve odors:** put lemon essential oil drops on a cotton ball and stuff cotton balls into athletic shoes or add a few drops to a diaper pail.

- Add a drop of lemon essential oil to the final rinse cycle on laundry day to make your laundry smell like fresh lemons.

- Lemon essential oil is a terrific grease remover. Dilute in a carrier oil and skin test before using on grime from your hands, as well as tools, dishes, and assorted household items.

- Lemon essential oil is a whiz at removing tree sap and the residue of glues from labels. Apply neat to objects or slightly diluted in a carrier oil.

- **Non-toxic wood cleaner:** add a few drops of lemon essential oil to some olive oil to make a wood cleaner and furniture polish without wax.[63]

- **For oily or greasy hair:** add 3 to 4 drops lemon essential oil to wet hands, apply to freshly washed hair, then rinse. This treatment reduces the need for frequent shampooing and adds shine to boot.

- **For an effective mosquito repellent:** mix lemon essential oil with a carrier oil (such as virgin coconut oil or jojoba oil) and rub over your skin to repel mosquitoes, who hate the smell. Citrus oils increase photosensitivity so please avoid the sun for at least 60 minutes after application.

- **To heal bug bites:** apply two drops diluted lemon essential oil directly to the bite and lightly rub. Do this two times during the day. Remember lemon essential oil increases photosensitivity.

- Carry a small vial of diluted lemon essential oil with you and rub a drop between your palms and fingers to sanitize your hands after using a public bathroom. You can premix a few drops of lemon essential oil in a small bottle of aloe vera gel and it will be a sanitizer for you. Be conscious of the photosensitivity of your hands after use.

- Lemon essential oil is also useful for treating stuffiness. Inhale the aroma of 2 to 3 drops of diluted lemon essential oil rubbed between your palms to clear nasal passages and sinuses.

- **For insomnia:** using a drop or 2 of lemon essential oil on a tissue or cloth and placed inside your pillowcase ensures good sleep and helps people that suffer from insomnia. (Oil may stain certain fabrics.)

- Use lemon essential oil for strong, healthy, and shiny hair and to eliminate dandruff. Add a few drops to your shampoo or conditioner and rinse.

---

63 "33 Awesome Uses of Lemon Essential Oil," www.beforeitsnews.com/selfsufficiency/2014 /uses-of-lemon-essential-oil.

Cautions

Lemon essential oil is powerfully astringent and antiseptic. Because it can cause skin irritation if used by sensitive individuals in dilutions exceeding 5 percent, it should not be applied undiluted to skin. Five drops or less of lemon essential oil should be added to 1 tsp. of a carrier oil. If you use diluted lemon essential oil directly on your skin, stay out of direct sunlight for at least 12 to 24 hours and apply a sunscreen before venturing outdoors. Sunscreens do have chemicals in them, so choose the ones with the least harmful ingredients.

Blends Well With

Lavender, rose, neroli, sandalwood, geranium, lemongrass, vetiver, rosemary, marjoram, ylang-ylang, and tea tree essential oils.

Supernatural Uses

Longevity, purification, love, friendship.

- Place a 1" piece of cloth which contains a drop of lemon essential oil beneath your visitor's chair and the friendship will be permanent.

- Wash used amulets, magical objects, and other second-hand jewelry in lemon essential oil and water to remove any negative vibrations.

- Use a drop or two of lemon essential oil on stationery and cards to enhance friendship.

- After a break-up or separation, use the lemon essential oil spray to purify the space and create room for a new love.

5: Bergamot

Bergamot is a small plant that produces a type of citrus fruit. Oil taken from the peel of the fruit is used to make the essential oil. It has been alleged that Christopher Columbus brought the very first tree with him from the Canary Islands to Spain and Italy.

Others claim Arab traders brought it from China. Bergamot oil was used in teas, perfumes, and healing and was a very valuable commodity during the fifteenth and sixteenth centuries. Twining made the first Earl Grey blend tea using bergamot essential oil as a flavoring.[64]

Its name originates from:

Latin: *Citrus bergamia, Mentha citrata*	**French:** *Bergamote*
	English: *Bergamot, orange mint*
Spanish: *Bergamota*	**Element:** *Air*
Gender: *Masculine*	**Ruling Planet:** *Mercury*

Property Description

Analgesic, stimulant, diuretic, antiseptic, antidepressant, deodorant, antitumoral, tonic, vermifuge, analgesic, febrifuge, cicatrisant, sedative, antibiotic.

Benefits

Relieves urinary tract infections, boosts liver functions, helps with the spleen and stomach, helps reduce oily skin, curtails acne, helps to clear up psoriasis, eczema, and cold sores, relieves depression, alleviates tension and fear.

Background

Originally native to tropical Asia, bergamot *(Citrus bergamia)* is now extensively cultivated in the south of Italy, in the Calabria region. It was named for an Italian city, Bergamot, where the essential oil was originally grown and sold. The Italians have used bergamot in natural medicine for years, in particular for fevers. It is also grown today in Tunisia, the Ivory Coast, Algeria, and Morocco.

Bergamot essential oil is obtained from the cold expression of the peel of nearly ripe fruit of the bergamot tree.[65] The small fruit tree produces round, very bitter, inedible (raw) fruit. The fruit resembles a miniature orange. Bergamot essential oil has a citrus-like aroma with a spicy undertone.

---

64   "What Is Bergamot Flavoring?" www.gardenandflowers.com/facts_7705251_bergamot -flavoring.html.

65   Dean Coleman, "Essential Oil Dictionary," www.deancoleman.org/essentialref.htm.

Recent Italian research has shown that bergamot essential oil has a wide variety of uses medicinally and in culinary dishes. Bergamot essential oil is useful for digestive difficulties, stress, infectious wounds, as an insect repellent, and for cystitis. Bergamot oil can also be used to treat depression, stress, tension, fear, hysteria, infection (all types including skin), anorexia, psoriasis, eczema, and for general convalescence. It also has superb antiseptic qualities that are useful for skin complaints such as acne, oily skin, eczema, psoriasis, and can also be used on cold sores, chicken pox, and wounds.

Bergamot essential oil is also helpful for respiratory problems, skin diseases, mouth and urinary tract infections. It has been used since the sixteenth century as a remedy for fever and as an antiseptic.[66] It is also renowned for being used as the secret flavoring in Earl Grey tea.[67]

Bergamot essential oil has helped with SAD (Seasonal Affected Disorder). If you are generally feeling just a bit off, lacking in self-confidence, reticent, or shy, you can diffuse or inhale bergamot essential oil for relief.

Bergamot essential oil has been shown to have a powerful effect on stimulating the liver, stomach, and spleen, demonstrating antiseptic qualities for urinary tract infections and inflammations such as cystitis.[68]

COMMON USES FOR BERGAMOT ESSENTIAL OIL

- Inhale or diffuse a few drop of bergamot essential oil to reduce anxiety.

- Psoriasis has been treated by applying the bergamot essential oil directly to the skin and then shining long-wave ultraviolet (UV) light on the affected area.[69] (Do not try at home. Hire a professional Aromatherapist skilled in this technique.)

---

66   Sharon Falsetto, "Bergamot Essential Oil," www.aromatherapylibrary.com /bergamotessentialoilprofile.html.

67   www.arborteas.com/organic-earl-grey-black-tea.html.

68   "Essential Oils and Blends," www.aromarakesh.com/essential.htm.

69   "Bergamot," www.webmd.com/vitamins-supplements/ingredientmono-142 –bergamot.aspx?activeingredientid=142&activeingredientname=bergamot.

- Use in a diffuser or inhaler to lift a dark mood, reduce anxiety, jittery nerves, nervous tension, and stress.

- Used as a spray mixed with water, bergamot oil promotes sleep. Add 10 drops bergamot to 1 oz. water. Shake well and spray on pillow before bed.

- Inhaled or diffused, a few drops of bergamot essential oil refreshes the senses, improves mental alertness, balances the nervous system, fights infections, and promotes illness recovery.

- Used in a diffuser, it can help a person overcome a smoking habit by diverting the impulse to smoke and regulate appetite.

- Loss or grief can be helped by diffusing bergamot and lavender essential oils mixed together.

- Use 10 drops in a bath to help cool off a fever. You can use 2 T of almond or coconut milk to help disperse the oils.

- Bergamot essential oil can help to regulate appetite when 3 to 4 drops are diffused.

- For a holiday treat, sprinkle drops of bergamot, myrrh, frankincense, and cinnamon bark essential oils on your holiday decorations to give them a festive scent.

- **For a super uplifting bath, mix bergamot essential oil with any of these oils:** clary sage, geranium, melissa, or frankincense. Use one or two oils, 10 to 15 drops total.

Cautions

Bergamot essential oil is highly phototoxic and should only be stored in dark bottles in dark places to protect it from sunlight because it can become poisonous if exposed to sunlight.[70] Stay out of the sun for at least 8 to 12 hours after it is applied or rubbed (diluted) onto the skin.

---

70 Rendering the skin susceptible to damage (as sunburn or blisters) upon exposure to light and especially ultraviolet light.

Do not use in cases of severe liver problems, and check with your doctor if you are taking medications for liver disease. Do not use when pregnant or nursing. Bergamot essential oil is a possible skin irritant. Discontinue use at least two weeks prior to surgery. Test a small area for sensitivity and be sure to dilute it well.

Blends Well With

Clary sage, frankincense, black pepper, geranium, sandalwood, orange, rosemary, vetiver, and ylang-ylang essential oils. It is particularly complementary with other citrus oils.

Supernatural Uses

Used to elevate the spirit, clarify the mind, assist with confidence-building, and inner strength. Bergamot essential oil helps to overcome disempowerment, victim consciousness, despondency, and helps to connect to one's higher self, highest calling, and inner purpose.

- Place several bergamot essential oil drops on a 1" cloth square and slip into your wallet or purse to build confidence.

- A few drops of bergamot essential oil can be used in rituals for attracting success and casting spells.

- Add bergamot essential oil to a diffuser to help you stay connected to life's purpose and meaning.

- Place 1 or 2 drops of bergamot essential oil on a 1" piece of cloth to protect yourself from being a victim or attracting people who want to use you.

6: Peppermint

Peppermint is a cross between two types of mint: water mint and spearmint. It grows plentifully—almost like a weed—throughout Europe and North America. Peppermint essential oil is used as a popular remedy for nausea, indigestion, cold symptoms, headaches, muscle and nerve pain, stomach problems, and intestinal conditions such as irritable bowel syndrome. Cooks have enjoyed the flavor and fragrance of peppermint in main courses, salads, and desserts for centuries.

Its name originates from:

Latin: *Mentha x piperita*	**French:** *menthe poivre*
Spanish: *menta*	**English:** *Peppermint, brandy mint, lammint*
Gender: *Masculine*	
Element: *Fire*	**Ruling Planet:** *Mercury*

Property Description

Analgesic, antispasmodic, antipyretic, stimulant, carminative, stomach tonic.

Benefits

Reduces stomachaches, freshens breath, relieves headaches, improves mental focus, clears respiratory tract, boosts energy, releases tight muscles, relieves nerve pain, lessens toothaches, and reduces fever.

Oddly enough, peppermint essential oil is also used in construction and plumbing to test for the tightness of pipes and disclose leaks by its odor.[71]

COMMON USES FOR PEPPERMINT ESSENTIAL OIL

- **To relieve a stomachache:** massage several drops of peppermint essential oil diluted with a carrier oil on your abdomen. Rub in a clockwise motion.

- Place a drop of peppermint essential oil on wrists, or inhale to soothe motion sickness or general nausea. Dilute according to your skin sensitivity.

- Use peppermint essential oil diluted in a carrier oil to massage and soothe an aching back, sore muscles, and melt away tension headaches.

- Apply diluted peppermint essential oil topically to relieve pain associated with fibromyalgia and myofascial pain syndrome. (One

---

71 Michele Booster, "Uses of Peppermint Oil Part 2," balancespaboca.com/part-2–uses-peppermint-oil.

study found that peppermint essential oil, eucalyptus essential oil, and capsaicin mixtures may be helpful.)[72]

- Inhaling diffused peppermint essential oil can unclog your sinuses and offer relief for scratchy throats.

- Diffused or inhaled as a steam, a few drops of peppermint essential oil can act as an expectorant and may provide the relief you need for colds, cough, sinusitis, asthma, and bronchitis.

- Apply a few drops of peppermint essential oil mixed with lavender essential oil and a carrier oil to achy joints to cool muscles like an ice, while you stay warm.

- Inhale peppermint essential oil to stave off the munchies. If you don't have a diffuser with you at dinnertime, apply a couple drops to your temples or chest, or take a couple of deep sniffs from the bottle. (You can easily make a portable inhaler to use as an appetite suppressant.) The aroma helps curb your appetite.

- **For an energy boost:** take a few whiffs of peppermint essential oil. It will perk you up on long road trips, in school, or times when you need a natural jolt of energy. Dilute and rub in your palms to sniff for a picker-upper.

- Diffused, 2 to 3 drops of peppermint essential oil may improve focus and concentration.

- Add 2 to 3 drops of peppermint essential oil to your regular shampoo and conditioner to stimulate the scalp and help remove dandruff.

- Inhaled or diffused, peppermint essential oil can relax muscles in your nasal passages and can help clear out the congestion and pollen during allergy season.

---

72 Josh Axe, MD, "Top 25 Uses of Peppermint Oil Uses and Benefits" draxe.com/peppermint-oil-uses-benefits/.

- Diffusing peppermint essential oil mixed with clove bud essential oil and eucalyptus essential oil can also reduce seasonal allergy symptoms.

- Inhale diluted peppermint essential oil to help curb your appetite by triggering a sense of fullness.

Cautions

Do not use in the first four months of pregnancy. In general, it is best to not use peppermint essential oil on children under three. Bronchial and respiratory stress can occur in infants and adults by using too strong a mixture on chest and nasal areas. Never apply undiluted peppermint essential oil to feet or on children under age twelve. Peppermint essential oil contains menthol and as such may result in dizziness and nausea if inhaled at too strong a dose. People with gallbladder disease, severe liver damage, gallstones, and chronic heartburn should avoid intake of peppermint essential oil. According to NAHA.org, peppermint essential oil should be used with caution. Doses of menthol over 1 g/Kg b.w. may be deadly.[73]

Blends Well With

Basil, benzoin, black pepper, eucalyptus, geranium, grapefruit, lavender, lemon, marjoram, cedarwood, ravensara, rosemary, and tea tree essential oils.

Supernatural Uses

Purification, love, sleep, healing, psychic powers.

- A drop of diluted peppermint essential oil worn on the wrist can ward off negative thoughts and energy about people.

- Sniffed or inhaled peppermint essential oil encourages a magical and dream-filled sleep.

- Drops of peppermint essential oil on a cloth beneath the pillow bring on dreams of the future.

---

73 NAHA Safety Note for Peppermint Essential Oil. www.naha.org/explore-aromatherapy /about-aromatherapy/most-commonly-used-essential-oils.

- Drops of peppermint essential oil diluted and rubbed lightly on furniture wards off evil. (Test first.)

- Enhance your psychic powers by diffusing a few drops of peppermint essential oil.

- The Roman author and naturalist Pliny the Elder wrote that peppermint "excites love."[74] As such, peppermint essential oil can be added to a love potion.

- Place 2 drops peppermint essential oil on a small 1" cloth and place in the wallet for prosperity.

7: Eucalyptus

Australian aboriginals have used oil-containing eucalyptus leaf infusions as a traditional medication for body pains, fever, sinus congestions, and colds for centuries. As early as the 1880s, surgeons had begun using eucalyptus essential oil as an antiseptic during operations.

Its name originates from:

Latin: *Eucalyptus globulus or Eucalyptus Radiata*	**French:** *Eucalypytus*
Spanish: *Eucalipto*	**English:** *Eucalyptus, blue gum tree, stringy bark tree*
Gender: *Feminine*	**Ruling Planet:** *Moon*
Element: *Water*	

Property Description

It works a lot like tea tree oil. It is favored as a general cure-all. Expectorant, antimicrobial, antiviral, antibacterial, antifungal.

---

74   www.aromatherapyinstitute.com/view_article.php?id=57.

Benefits

Respiratory and sinus infections, rheumatism relief, sore muscles, coughs, inflammation, asthma, bronchitis, antiseptic, insect repellent, and treatment option for wounds, burns, and ulcers.

Background

There are over five hundred different species of eucalyptus growing and cultivated. Because of the wide variety, it is important to know which species of this essential oil you are using. Here are a few common ones:

1. *Eucalyptus polybractea*—called the blue mallee, or blue-leaved mallee tree.

2. *Eucalyptus globulus*—best known and most used for eucalyptus essential oils.

3. *Eucalyptus radiata*—commonly known as the narrow-leaved peppermint tree.

4. *Eucalyptus citriodora*—called the lemon-scented gum, the principal constituent of the oil is citronella, used for industrial and perfume purposes.[75]

Early European explorers to Australia first saw eucalypts, but no botanical collections are known to have been made until 1777 during Captain James Cook's third expedition when botanist David Nelson collected a eucalypt on Bruny Island, southern Tasmania, and took it back to England. French botanist Charles-Louis L'Héritier coined a generic name from the Greek roots *eu* and *calyptos*, meaning "well" and "covered" in reference to the operculum of the flower bud.[76]

---

75 "Organic Eucalyptus Oil," eucalyptusoil.com/eucalyptus-oils/eucalyptus-citriadora.

76 "L'Heritier de Brutelle, Charles Louis, (1746–1800)," Encyclopedia of Australian Science, www .eoas.info/biogs/P005304b.htm.

In 1948, the United States also officially registered eucalyptus oil as an insecticide and miticide (kills mites and ticks).[77]

Eucalyptus essential oil is also popularly used as a fragrance in perfumes and cosmetics, and is found in toothpastes, mouthwashes, cough drops, ointments, and lozenges. It is commonly mixed with other oils to make it more easily absorbed by the skin.

Although similar in properties to tea tree essential oil, eucalyptus essential oil is a bit more effective for treating bronchial and respiratory infections while tea tree essential oil is better for topical antiseptic applications due to its skin-friendly qualities. I think having both covers your bases.

There are several different ways to use eucalyptus essential oil, including aromatically, topically, or internally. For instance, it can be applied to skin diluted in a carrier oil such as virgin coconut oil, jojoba, or sweet almond oil. Start with a 2 drops added to 1 to 3 tsp. of carrier oil, increasing the amount of eucalyptus oil as needed.

COMMON USES FOR EUCALYPTUS ESSENTIAL OIL

- Apply a drop of eucalyptus essential oil to a cotton ball and sniff it several times a day to heal mucus membranes and treat allergies and asthma.

- Add a few drops of refreshing eucalyptus essential oil to water or a nebulizer as steam therapy for coughs, colds, or sinus inflammation and congestion.

- Use a few drops of diluted eucalyptus essential oil in your bath water.

- **To decongest and heal a respiratory infection:** diffuse 4 drops of eucalyptus essential oil for 20 to 30 minutes three times a day.

- Apply diluted eucalyptus essential oil to the soles of your feet to help with a cold, cough, or congestion (5 drops eucalyptus essential oil to 1 tsp. carrier oil).

- Dilute 4 drops eucalyptus essential oil in 1 T carrier oil and then rub on the chest, feet, back, neck, and down the spine for relief of colds, congestion, or fever.

---

77   "Cosmetic and Personal Care Formulations," naturalingredient.org/?p=1946.

- Put a drop or 2 of diluted eucalyptus essential oil on a blister to alleviate the swelling and to disinfect the area.

- Steam out a cold with 5 drops each of eucalyptus essential oil, thyme, tea tree, and lavender essential oils.

- To help ease a cough, add 3 drops marjoram essential oil to the above steam mix. Add 4 drops frankincense essential oil instead if the cough has settled.

- Try eucalyptus essential oil diluted and dispersed in a sponge bath to reduce fevers.

- **Make an antiviral spray:** mix 10 drops eucalyptus essential oil with 10 drops tea tree essential oil, 4 drops of thyme essential oil, and 6 drops lavender essential oil in 10 oz. clean water. Use it as an air spray for the home or office. Shake well before spraying.

- Eucalyptus essential oil can be effective as an antiseptic on herpes and shingles. Modify your dilution beginning with 2 to 3 drops per teaspoon and make sure your carrier oil is pure.

- Concentration can be focused by inhaling a few diluted drops or by diffusing eucalyptus essential oil.

- Eucalyptus essential oil can also be used in the bath, diluted, or blended as a massage oil—it can provide benefits for arthritis, asthma, congestion, colds, headaches, sinusitis, fatigue, and muscle aches and pains.

- Use a few drops of eucalyptus essential oil to speed up the healing of wounds and skin ulcers. Add a few drops to an antiseptic or therapeutic cream or lotion for pain relief.

- Use diluted eucalyptus essential oil on your skin for relief of insect bites or wounds, but be very careful when doing so. Use only a drop at a time.

- Eucalyptus essential oil can be used as a wash to cleanse wounds. Mix a few drops in clean, warm water, and use a sterile cloth on wounds.

- Add 10 drops eucalyptus essential oil per oz. of shampoo to help maintain beautiful hair and a healthy scalp.

- To disinfect surfaces, add 10 to 20 drops of eucalyptus essential oil to a spray bottle and add warm water. (Add a few drops of lemon essential oil if you like.) Using this eucalyptus essential oil spray on bedding and mattresses can help eliminate bed bugs.

- Add eucalyptus essential oil to your detergent when you launder your sheets to help eliminate bed bugs and dust mites. (You can also freeze your sheets to kill those mites.)

Cautions

Eucalyptus essential oil is strong and should not be used on babies or children under two years, even diluted. It has been known to cause respiratory problems in young children.

The maximum concentration when mixed with a carrier oil should be 20 percent. (To achieve this ratio, mix 20 drops of eucalyptus essential oil to 1 tsp. of carrier oil for short-term use.)

Blends Well With

Tea tree, lavender, thyme, lemongrass, lemon, basil, bergamot, cedarwood, ginger, pink grapefruit, marjoram, orange, peppermint, and rosemary essential oils.

Supernatural Uses

Eucalyptus essential oil clears the air and is used for healing physical and emotional issues that are blocked or stuck. It is used for protection, good health, and warding off intruders.

- Place a few drops of eucalyptus essential oil on a small piece of cloth and place beneath your pillow to ward off colds or low resistance.

- Place a few drops of eucalyptus essential oil on a 1" cloth square and sniff it in times of emotional upset or in the presence of emotional triggers.

- Diffuse eucalyptus essential oil during meditation when you want to break through nagging issues.

- Diffuse eucalyptus essential oil at the new year or on your birthday when you want to make positive changes in your life.

- Place a few drops of eucalyptus essential oil on a talisman and carry it as protection against unwanted interlopers.

8: Roman Chamomile

Roman chamomile was one of the nine sacred oils of the Saxons.[78] The word "chamomile" (sometimes spelled "camomile" and generally pronounced with a short *i*) is derived from Greek—*chamos* (ground) and *melos* (apple), referring to the fact that the plant grows low to the ground and the fresh blooms have a pleasing apple scent. The Spaniards called it *manzanilla*, ("little apple"), and gave the same name to one of their sherries which was flavored with this aromatic plant.[79]

Its name originates from:

Latin: *Anthemis nobilis or Chamaemelum nobile*	**French:** *Camomille romaine*
Spanish: *Manzanilla romana*	**English:** *Chamomile, English chamomile, garden chamomile, ground apple, sweet chamomile, whig plant*
Gender: *Masculine*	
Element: *Water*	**Ruling Planet:** *Sun*

Property Description

Anti-inflammatory, analgesic, nervine, relaxant, sedative.

Benefits

Helps decrease gas (flatulence), relaxes muscles, treats hay fever, inflammation, rheumatism, muscle spasms, PMS, menstrual disorders, insomnia, ulcers, gastrointestinal disorders, hemorrhoids, nervousness, joint stiffness, and muscular aches and pains.

---

78 "Plants in the Medieval World," www.psumedievalgarden.com/sacred_saxon_herbs.html.

79 "Chamomille," www.herbs-info.com/chamomile.html.

It also relieves dry, itchy skin, puffiness, and some allergic conditions. Known as a skin aid, it can heal blisters and improve elasticity and tissue strength. It has even been used to lighten fair hair.

Background

The early Egyptians, Greeks, and Romans reportedly used chamomile widely for its gentle, healing qualities. The English used it in the pot for stews, and as mentioned on the previous page, the Spanish used it to flavor their vintages of sherry.

If you step on the growing plant, chamomile releases a strong and potent airborne smell. Legend has it that nothing contributes so much to the health of a garden as a number of chamomile plants dispersed about.

If one of the other plants is drooping and sickly, it is said to recover if you place a chamomile plant or a cutting near it. Its fame has been recounted in print by William Shakespeare and in Beatrix Potter's *Tale of Peter Rabbit*:

> Mrs. Rabbit put Peter to bed, made some chamomile tea, and gave a dose of it to her unruly son. "One table-spoonful to be taken at bed time."[80] Just what was this elixir that calmed our favorite woodland renegade?

Before WWII, chamomile was largely cultivated in Belgium, France, Saxony (a region of Germany), and England. Of all the varieties, the English flower heads are considered the most valuable for distillation of the oil. During the war, the price of English chamomile became exorbitant.

There are several types of chamomile available as an essential oil. I am recommending Roman chamomile essential oil in our primary palette. Several varieties are grown in England, Morocco, and western Europe.

If you want to test the difference for yourself, check a pile of dried chamomile flowers and you will be able to distinguish the Roman from the German by splitting the flower receptacle open down the middle. If the receptacle is solid, it is Roman; if hollow, it is German.

---

80   "Chamomille," www.motherearthliving.com/health-and-wellness/chamomile-herb
    -zmaz91djzgoe.aspx.

COMMON USES FOR ROMAN CHAMOMILE ESSENTIAL OIL

- Roman chamomile essential oil can be applied topically, as a compress, in the bath, through direct inhalation, or a few drops in a diffuser.

- Add a few drops of Roman chamomile essential oil to bath water before bedtime to bring calm, peaceful sleep.

- Diffuse Roman chamomile essential oil or apply several drops diluted to the soles of feet to reduce fever and calm frayed nerves.

- **For an anti-inflammatory:** mix together 3 drops Roman chamomile essential oil, 3 drops helichrysum essential oil, 2 drops cedarwood essential oil, and 2 drops of yarrow essential oil in 1 oz. carrier oil and apply topically as needed.

- **A gentle bath for all ages:** 2 drops Roman chamomile essential oil, 2 drops lavender essential oil in warm bath water. Disperse and dilute with almond, coconut, or rice milk.

- For an adult bath or massage, add 10 drops Roman chamomile essential oil to a warm bath for relaxation. Disperse and dilute with almond, coconut, or rice milk.

- Diluted with a carrier oil, it can be massaged in or with a few drops placed in a warm cloth, used as a compress for headaches.

- Diffuse a few drops of fragrant Roman chamomile essential oil to ease headaches and nervous tension.

- Add 1 or 2 drops of Roman chamomile essential oil to your favorite moisturizer, shampoo, or conditioner to promote youthful looking skin and hair.

- Add drops of Roman chamomile essential oil in a steam bath and inhale it for sinus inflammation, hay fever, sore throat, ear inflammation, and pain.

- **For supple skin:** add Roman chamomile essential oil to your face or body lotion, or use a very small amount of essential oil mixed with virgin coconut oil.

- **For a calming and restorative salve:** combine ½ C pure virgin coconut oil with ¼ C beeswax and heat on low or medium heat until mixed. Be careful not to burn the mixture. During the cooling process stir in 15 drops each of Roman chamomile and lavender essential oils.

- Adding a few drops of Roman chamomile essential oil, mixed with 1 tsp. of carrier oil to bath water can ease inflammation of the skin and soothe a sunburn.

- **For restful sleep:** combine witch hazel, 10 drops each of Roman chamomile essential oil and lavender essential oil, and 5 drops orange essential oil in a 4 oz. spray bottle. Shake well. Spray on linens before for bed for more restful sleep.

Cautions
Avoid using Roman chamomile essential oil if you are pregnant or breastfeeding.[81]

Roman chamomile essential oil can cause an allergic reaction in people who are sensitive to ragweed, chrysanthemums, marigolds, daisies, and others.[82] If you have allergies, check with your healthcare provider before using Roman chamomile essential oil.

Blends Well With
Bergamot, clary sage, eucalyptus, geranium, grapefruit, lavender, lemon, neroli, rose, tea tree, and ylang-ylang essential oils.

Supernatural Uses
Roman chamomile essential oil brings love, money, purification, and sleep.

---

81 Dahlia Kelada, "Essential Oils to Avoid While Pregnant or Breastfeeding." mirvacu.com /uncategorized/essential-oils-to-avoid-while-pregnant-and-breastfeeding.

82 Natural Medicine Comprehensive Database. naturaldatabase.therapeuticresearch.com/nd /PrintVersion.aspx/roman_chamomile.

- Gamblers used to wash their hands with chamomile oil and water to ensure their money would return to them.[83]

- Sprinkled around a property, it can remove curses.

- Patted above a doorway it can provide protection and bring happiness to the inhabitants.

- A few drops on a 1" cloth square placed under a pillow bring a peaceful and calm night's sleep.

- A few drops on a 1" cloth and sniffed gently relieves tension and worry.

9: Frankincense

Frankincense was brought to Europe by the Crusaders. The *franc* in its name refers to the quality, not the French. Commonly known as *frankincense* to westerners, the resin is known as *olibanum*, in Arabic *al-lubān*, meaning "that which results from milking" or "the product resulting from milking the boswellia tree."[84]

Its name originates from:

Latin: *Boswellia carterii*	**French:** *Franc encens*
Spanish: *El incienso*	**English:** *Frankincense*
Gender: *Masculine*	**Ruling Planet:** *Sun*
Element: *Fire*	

Property Description

Anti-inflammatory, astringent, tonic, antiseptic, disinfectant, digestive, diuretic, expectorant, cicatrisant, carminative, cytophylactic, emenagogue, uterine, and vulnerary.

---

83 "The Magickal Properties of Herbs, Roots, Barks, Flowers, and Resins," www.themagickalcat .com/Articles.asp?ID=242.

84 "Frankincense," naturalingredient.org/wp/wp-content/uploads/Frankincense.pdf.

Benefits

Many bodily systems, including the digestive, respiratory, nervous, and excretory systems can be helped by frankincense essential oil. It aids the absorption of nutrients and strengthens the immune system.

Frankincense essential oil has been found useful for certain health conditions like rheumatoid arthritis, stomach ulcers, asthma, breaking up phlegm, and helping digestive disorders by stimulating gastric juices and bile production.[85]

The antiseptic qualities of this oil can help prevent bad breath, cavities, toothaches, mouth sores, and other infections.

Frankincense essential oil often regulates estrogen production in women and reduces the risk of post-menopausal tumor or cyst formation in the uterus (uterine cancer). It also can regulate the menstrual cycle of premenopausal women.[86]

Frankincense essential oil is being studied for its potential to treat cancer. Scientists have observed that there's an agent in this oil that not only stops cancer from spreading, but also induces cancerous cells to close themselves down. Immunologist Mahmoud Suhail is hoping to open a new chapter in the history of frankincense.

> "Cancer starts when the DNA code within the cell's nucleus becomes corrupted," Dr. Suhail says. "It seems frankincense has a re-set function. It can tell the cell what the right DNA code should be." [87]

In a series of clinical and laboratory studies over the last two decades, frankincense and myrrh have shown promise in addressing a number of common disorders. Frankincense has been investigated as a possible treatment for some cancers, ulcerative colitis, Crohn's disease, anxiety, and asthma, among other conditions. If these ancient remedies

---

85   Joseph Mercola MD, "Frankincense," articles.mercola.com/herbal-oils/frankincense-oil.aspx.

86   "Cosmetic and Personal Care Formulations," NaturalIngredient.com, http://naturalingredient .org/?p=1961.

87   Jeremy Howell, "Frankincense: Could It Be a Cure for Cancer?" news.bbc.co.uk/2/hi/middle _east/8505251.stm.

can indeed provide relief for the many patients who suffer from these potentially devastating illnesses, the great incense roads of antiquity may flourish once again.[88]

The concern among some in the scientific community is the presence of boswellic acid which is not present in frankincense essential oil, only in frankincense extracts, which contain 40 to 60 percent of boswellic acid. Robert Tisserand writes:

> [I]f you are looking for a natural substance to help prevent or treat cancer, frankincense oil should not be your first choice. Look instead to turmeric/curcumin, to cannabis/cannabinoids, to garlic/garlic oil, and to frankincense extract, which is sold in capsule form. Following that, I would consider essential oils of cinnamon bark, lemongrass, citronella, turmeric, orange, lemon and bergamot.[89]

My advice is to work with a qualified Aromatherapist before trying any of these methods.

Only time and research will tell us what the future of essential oils are in the cure for cancer. I am looking forward to seeing more results.

Background

Frankincense (commonly referred to as olibanum), *Boswellia carteri* comes from the *Boswellia* genus trees, particularly *Boswellia sacra* and *Boswellia carteri*.

After the milky white sap is extracted from the tree bark, it is allowed to harden for several days into a gum resin, after which it is scraped off in perfect tear-shaped droplets.

Frankincense is traditionally burned as incense and was charred and ground into a powder to produce the heavy kohl eyeliner used by ancient makeup artists and applied to upper class Egyptian women and royalty that classic artwork and Hollywood movies have portrayed.

---

88 Jennie Cohen, "A Wiseman's Cure: Frakincense and Myrrh," www.history.com/news/a-wise -mans-cure-frankincense-and-myrrh.

89 Robert Tisserand, "Frankincense Oil and Cancer in Perspective," tisserandinstitute.org /frankincense-oil-and-cancer-in-perspective.

When the resin is steam-distilled, it produces an aromatic essential oil with a bounty of benefits. In ancient Egypt, frankincense was revered as the sweat of the gods.[90]

Remarkably, frankincense resin is edible and is used in traditional medicines in Africa and Asia for digestion and healthy skin.[91] For internal consumption, it is recommended that frankincense be translucent, with no black or brown impurities. It is often light yellow with a (very) slight greenish tint. It is often chewed like gum but is stickier.

In Ayurvedic medicine frankincense (*Boswellia serrata*) is commonly referred to in India as "*dhoop*," and has been used for hundreds of years for treating arthritis, healing wounds, strengthening the female hormone system, and purifying the air.[92]

The Greek historian Herodotus was familiar with frankincense and knew it was harvested from trees in southern Arabia. He reported that the gum was dangerous to harvest because of the venomous snakes living in the trees. The method Arabs used to get around this problem was to burn the gum of the styrax tree letting off smoke that would drive the snakes away.

Recent studies have indicated that the worldwide frankincense tree populations are declining partly due to over-exploitation. Frequently tapped trees produce seeds that germinate at a rate of 16 percent while seeds of trees that had not been tapped germinate at a rate of more than 80 percent. In addition, burning, grazing, and attacks by the longhorn beetle have reduced the tree population to an unsafe level of potential extinction.[93] Only responsible farmers who are conscientious about preservation and use sustainable methods for growing and harvesting will keep this sacred tree alive for generations to come. As a general rule when using natural products, we should patronize those growers and manufacturers who practice sustainability.

---

90   Janet Hull, PhD, CN, "Frankincense—Is This an Ancient Hope Reborn," www.JanetHull.com, http://www.janethull.com/healthynews/blog/2014/05/frankincense-an-ancient-cure-for -cancer-re-born-2/.

91   "Frankincense Breu Resin Incense," mantraincense.bigcartel.com/product/mantra -frankincense.

92   "Frankincense (Dhoop)," www.mangalorespice.com/Products/Herbs—Aromatics-Aromatics /M-Spice/Frankincense-(Dhoop)/pid-3856277.aspx.

93   "Frankincense," naturalingredient.org/wp/wp-content/uploads/Frankincense.pdf.

COMMON USES FOR FRANKINCENSE ESSENTIAL OIL

- Frankincense essential oil can be used for relief from stings such as scorpion stings. Use 1 drop neat on the sting. Dilute if needed.

- Use as a wrinkle relief (night or day) cream by adding a few drops of frankincense essential oil to the base cream or lotion of your choice.

- Add frankincense essential oil to pure water and use as a toner or refresher. (You can add a drop or two of vodka to help it blend together.)

- Place a few drops of frankincense essential oil on your washcloth and run it over yourself during your final shower (warm) rinse. The steam will infuse the frankincense essential oil and you get the benefit of a quick and refreshing, frankincensed steam bath.

- If you want to enjoy a special indulgence, use frankincense essential oil in the bath and disperse it with almond, coconut, or rice milk. This breaks up the oil and spreads it out in the water. Epsom salts also works well for the same dispersion purpose.

- Treat dry skin by mixing a few drops of frankincense essential oil in a tsp. of carrier oil like sweet almond, pomegranate, or carrot oil and massage it onto your face.

- Treat wrinkles and the signs of aging by adding 2 drops of frankincense essential oil to your nightly moisturizing cream or lotion treatment. Add one to two drops of sandalwood essential oil for a richer treatment.

- Reduce the appearance of stretch marks and scars by mixing 2 drops of frankincense essential oil with 2 drops of lavender essential oil and 1 drop neroli essential oil in 1 T carrier oil and massage onto scar tissue.

- For a revitalizing face serum mix 2 drops of frankincense and 2 drops of lavender essential oils in 1 oz. of carrier oil. Massage into skin using an upward motion.

- Diffuse or inhale a few drops of frankincense essential oil directly to lift your mood.

- Mix a few drops of frankincense essential oil with double the drops of a carrier oil (jojoba is good) to strengthen hair roots.

- Speed up the healing of cuts, acne, insect bites, and boils. After doing a patch test for safety, use a small drop of diluted frankincense essential oil on the pimple or bite.

Cautions

Frankincense essential oil should not be used during pregnancy. Avoid using if the oil has oxidized.

Blends Well With

Lemon, orange, bergamot, lavender, myrrh, sandalwood, other citrus oils, black pepper, basil, geranium, melissa, and vetiver essential oils.

Supernatural Uses

Frankincense oil promotes acceptance, emotional balance and stability, offers protection, fortitude, courage and resolution; increases introspection, spiritual awareness, and inspiration; is an aid in meditative practices and prayer work.

- Frankincense essential oil can be used as an anointing oil used for ceremonies, rituals, and rites of passage.

- Diffuse for meditation to access awareness and inspiration.

- Honor ancestors by placing a drop of frankincense beneath their picture or near a keepsake.

- Amulets coated with frankincense essential oil can be used as protection.

10: Sandalwood

Also known by its nickname, "liquid gold," sandalwood is an evergreen tree native to southern Asia. The oil comes from the heartwood of the tree. Sandalwood was first recorded in

78 CE by Dioscorides in *De Materia Medica*, a book filled with descriptions of hundreds of plants and herbs. This book was used as the standard reference until some time in the seventeenth century.

Its name originates from:

Latin: *Santalum album*	**French:** *Bois de santal*
Spanish: *Sandalo*	**English:** *Sandalwood, white sandalwood, sandal, santal*
Gender: *Feminine*	
Element: *Water*	**Ruling Planet:** *Moon*

Property Description

Astringent, disinfectant, stimulant, tonic, antidepressant, antibacterial, antiviral, immune stimulant, antitumoral.

Benefits

Calming, grounding, stabilizing, sacred, aphrodisiac. Also helpful with skin repair, as a relaxant, and helpful for urogenital and pulmonary disorders, viral infections, cold sores, and herpes simplex.

Background

Sandalwood essential oil has a distinctive soft, warm, smooth, creamy, and milky precious-wood scent. It has been used for centuries and, among other sacred uses, it was used extensively to perfume the mortar and bricks from which ancient buildings, temples, and monuments were made.[94] True sandalwoods belong to the same botanical family as European mistletoe. Indian sandalwood (*Santalum album*) and Australian sandalwood (*Santalum spicatum*) head the list of desirable producers. It is ecologically important to distinguish between the different sandalwood essential oils on the market. The main source of true sandalwood, *Santalum album*, Indian sandalwood, is a protected species, and current demand for it cannot be adequately met. The genus *Santalum* has more than nineteen

---

94 "Egypt Under The Ethiopians" www.gutenberg.org/files/15663/15663–h/15663–h.htm #Page_314.

species. Some avaricious traders try to pawn off these other species as "the real deal" but they are not. Most of the substitute woods are substandard and lose their aroma quickly. It's probably best to stay with Indian sandalwood essential oil products as long as they are fairly traded and responsibly harvested by growers who renew their assets.

Similar plants in the same *Santalum* genus are grown in India, Nepal, Bangladesh, Pakistan, Sri Lanka, Australia, Indonesia, and Hawaii. Hawaiian sandalwood was also overharvested and is now rare and pricey. From the 1790s to the mid-1830s, the Hawaiian people harvested the sandalwood logs and exported them to China. The Chinese nicknamed the Hawaiian islands "Sandalwood Mountains."[95]

Santalum album trees in India are now owned by the government in order to monitor the illegal harvesting of the trees. The Indian government controls 75 percent of the total output of sandalwood in the world. The legal harvesting mandate is: a sandalwood tree should be at least fifteen years old before it is cut down. Sadly, illegal tree poaching is a recurring national problem; many trees get the axe well before their time, often in the dead of night, thus creating a product in the marketplace that is inferior.

Sandalwood has a proud and sacred four-thousand–year-old history. It has been featured in ancient Sanskrit and Chinese manuscripts. Sandalwood essential oil was used in countless religious rituals and many deities and temples were even carved from its soft wood to be fragrant icons and monuments.

Ancient Egyptians imported the wood and used it for medicines, embalming, and ritual burnings to venerate their gods.[96] Sandalwood essential oil was believed to promote spiritual practices, peaceful relaxation, openness, and grounding. It is still used in many funeral ceremonies to help the dead cross over and also as a comfort for the mourners. Historically it's been used in many initiation rites to open the disciple's mind when he is about to receive consecration.[97]

In Hinduism, sandalwood paste is central to various rituals and ceremonies. It is used to anoint religious utensils and to decorate the icons of the deities. Devotees apply it to

---

95 "Sandalwood Mountain," pbshawaii.org/ourproductions/sandalwood.htm/.

96 "Safety Assessment of Sandalwood Oil," www.sciencedirect.com/science/article/pii /S0278691507004309.

97 www.scents-of-earth.com/

their foreheads, necks, and chests as a purifying ritual. Only high priests are allowed to make the paste.[98]

In Buddhism it is one of the three incenses integral to sacred practice along with aloeswood (*Lignum aloes*) and cloves. Sandalwood is mentioned in various sutras of the Pāli canon in the Buddhist tradition.

The sandalwood scent is believed by some to transform one's desires, to maintain a person's focus while meditating, and to bring one closer to the divine. It is one of the most popular scents used for offerings.[99]

In the Tamil culture, sandalwood paste or powder is applied to the graves of Sufis as a mark of devotion and respect.[100]

Sandalwood is called *sukhar* in the Zoroastrian community and it is offered to the priests to keep the sacred fires burning which soothe and absorb the troubles of all humanity.[101]

COMMON USES FOR SANDALWOOD ESSENTIAL OIL

- Diffuse a few drops of sandalwood essential oil at bedtime to relax and de-stress before sleep.

- Apply several drops (2 to 4) of sandalwood essential oil on stressed locations, ankles, and wrists (patch test first).

- Directly inhale fumes of sandalwood essential oil from a drop-soaked cotton ball.

- Place a few drops of sandalwood essential oil in a bedside diffuser.

- 3 to 4 drops of sandalwood essential oil added to a vaporizer can be used as an effective aphrodisiac.

---

98   "What is Red Sandalwood?" jsrgroupsuncity.com, http://jsrgroupsuncity.com/admin/tiny _mce/plugins/filemanager/files/Red_sandalwood_Uses.pdf.

99   "Sandalwood," anandfoodproducts.com/sandal.php.

100   "Sandalwood," medlibrary.org/medwiki/Sandalwood.

101   Dastur Soli, "Dhala: Saga part 2—AVESTA," www.avesta.org/dhalla/saga2.htm.

- Use drops of sandalwood essential oil in a diffuser or make an inhaler to clear bronchitis, coughs, chest infections, asthma, irritability, nervous tension, stress.

- To totally bring about relaxation, place a few drops of sandalwood essential oil in a vaporizer or diffuser.

- Use a few drops of sandalwood essential oil in a vaporizer to ward off bugs like an insect repellant.

- Use a few drops of sandalwood essential oil mixed with a carrier oil, and almond, rice, or coconut milk in bathwater to alleviate bladder infections, scar tissue, improve eczema and stretch marks.

- Add a few drops of sandalwood essential oil to your favorite lotion or cream to assist with chapped, dry, or inflamed skin. Sandalwood essential oil has wonderful moisturizing and hydrating properties, which are great for antiaging skin care. For wrinkles, massage 1 or 2 drops of sandalwood essential oil directly into the area of concern, lightly diluted with a moisturizer or carrier oil of your choice.

- Mix drops of sandalwood essential oil into carrier oil for a skin-softening effect for neck and face.

- Use diluted sandalwood essential oil mixed with 1 oz. pure water as a toner for aiding oily skin.

- For an at-home facial, fill a large bowl with steaming water, then apply 1 or 2 drops of diluted sandalwood essential oil (make sure you do a patch test first) to your face and cover head with a towel. Place your face over the steaming water for 5 to 10 minutes. Your skin will feel nourished and rejuvenated.

- To help restore moisture and give hair a silky shine, apply 1 or 2 drops of sandalwood essential oil to wet hair.

- Two drops of diluted sandalwood essential oil placed directly into palms and rubbed together then inhaled will lessen tension and balance emotions. Diffuse for the same results.

Cautions

Breastfeeding mothers and young children should avoid using sandalwood essential oil.[102] The oil can cause an allergic skin reaction in certain individuals, so it is important to patch test on a small area of skin first.

Anyone with a medical condition such as liver disorder and cancer should also take extra precaution using the oil.[103]

Blends Well With

Bergamot, black pepper, geranium, lavender, palo santo, myrrh, rose, vetiver, and ylang-ylang essential oils.

Supernatural Uses

Protection, full moon rituals, wishes come true, healing, exorcism, past lives.

Sandalwood essential oil awakens sensuality, invokes calmness and deep relaxation. It opens cellular memory of past life experiences.

- Diffuse a few drops with lavender essential oil to conjure spirits.

- Diffuse or mix a few diluted drops with frankincense essential oil for full moon rituals and anointing.

- Write your wish on a 3" piece of cloth and drop sandalwood essential oil on it. Place under your pillow and visualize it coming true.

- Place a few drops of diluted sandalwood essential oil on a cotton ball, inhale to help recall past life experiences.

---

102 Joseph Mercola MD, "Sandalwood Oil: Calming and Beyond," articles.mercola.com/herbal -oils/sandalwood-oil.aspx.

103 Ibid.

- Sandalwood essential oil can be used in many bereavement ceremonies to help with the crossing over process and to ease the loss of mourners.

- Sandalwood essential oil is also used in many forms of initiation rites to open the disciple's mind to receive consecration.

11: Thyme

This perennial herb and member of the mint family, thyme (*Thymus vulgaris*) has a number of outstanding healing properties due to the herb's powerful essential oils.

Its name originates from:

Latin: *Thymus vulgaris*	**French:** *Thym*
Spanish: *Tomillo*	**English:** *Common thyme, garden thyme*
Gender: *Feminine*	
Element: *Water*	**Ruling Planet:** *Venus*

Property Description

Antibacterial, antiviral, stimulant, antispasmodic, bactericide, parasiticide, hypotensive, expectorant, emenagogue.

Benefits

Used to relieve and treat problems like gout, arthritis, wounds, bites, sores, water retention, menstrual and menopausal problems, nausea and fatigue, respiratory problems (colds), skin conditions (oily skin and scars), athlete's foot, hangovers, and even depression by diffusing or inhaling the scent of thyme essential oil.

In 2010 Professor Yiannis Samaras and Dr. Effimia Eriotou, from the Technological Educational Institute of Ionian Islands, Greece, tested the antimicrobial activity of eight plant essential oils.[104] Their research concluded that thyme essential oil was the

---

104 "Use Essential Oils to Fight Superbug," www.massagemag.com/use-essential-oils-to-fight-superbugs-7130.

most effective because it was able to almost completely eliminate bacteria within sixty minutes.[105]

In a study presented at the Society for General Microbiology's spring conference in Edinburgh 2014, it was emphasized that certain essential oils may be efficient and affordable alternatives to antibiotics in the battle against resistant bacteria.[106]

Among the essential oils tested in the study, cinnamon essential oil and thyme essential oil were found to be the most successful combatants against various *Staphylococcus* species, including the dreaded MRSA.

Researchers said that these oils can help lower antibiotic use and minimize the formation of new resistant strains of microorganisms.[107]

Essential oils could be a cheap and effective alternative to antibiotics and potentially used to combat drug-resistant hospital superbugs, according to research presented at the Society for General Microbiology's in Edinburgh.[108]

The benefits of thyme essential oil have been recognized for thousands of years in Mediterranean countries.

Today, among the many producers of thyme essential oil, France, Morocco, and Spain emerge as the primary suppliers. We refer to the chemotype thyme ct linalool as our essential oil of choice.

Background

Thyme was an herb and an oil used by the Egyptians for embalming. It was believed to help the dead person cross over into eternal life.

---

105 "Essential Oils to Fight Superbugs," www.sciencedaily.com/releases/2010/03/100330210942
    .htm; www.sciencedaily.com/releases/2010/03/100330210942.htm.

106 "Essential Oils for the Non Believer," www.rainshadowlabs.com/Essential-Oils-for-the-Non
    -Believer_b_217.html.

107 Ibid.

108 "Essential Oils to Fight Superbugs," sciencedaily.com.

The Greeks burned thyme outside their temples as purification of the space. The word "thyme" is thought to come from the Greek word *thumos* meaning "smoke" because of temple purification rituals.

The Greeks also burned the herb before games and physical contests because it was thought to invoke courage. Virgil cited it as a cure for exhaustion.[109]

The Romans were very fond of thyme because it was purported to be an antidote to poison. Many emperors consumed it or drank a drop of the oil before feasting to prevent poisoning.

Thyme was a visible badge of honor in the Middle Ages. Knights setting off to battle wore sprigs of it on their armor for courage and protection.

Young women were encouraged on St Luke's Day to sleep with thyme under their pillows as a love potion so they would dream of the man they would marry.

Thyme has many magical attributes including from the Victorians who believed a patch of thyme found in the woods signified the presence of fairies.[110] It has been called the superstar of a garden.

Common Uses for Thyme Essential Oil

- Diffuse thyme essential oil to stimulate the mind, strengthen the memory, improve concentration and calm the nerves.

- Use drops of thyme essential oil as a treatment for the scalp by adding a few drops to shampoos and other hair products to stimulate the scalp and prevent hair loss.

- Thyme essential oil can help tone aged skin and prevent acne outbreaks. Apply carefully and dilute in a carrier oil before applying topically.

- Adding a few drops to your mouthwash, thyme essential oil can be used to fight bad breath and reduce gum inflammation.

---

109   "A Brief History of Thyme," www.history.com/news/hungry-history/a-brief-history-of-thyme.

110   "Thyme History," www.ourherbgarden.com/herb-history/thyme.html.

- Used as a repellant, a few drops of thyme essential oil can keep insects and parasites like mosquitoes, fleas, lice, and moths away. Dilute with a carrier oil if rubbing directly onto skin.

- **To relieve pain:** mix 3 drops of thyme essential oil with 2 tsp. of sesame oil. Use this mixture as a massage oil and apply on the abdominal area to relieve pain. The same mixture of thyme essential oil may also be used as a massage oil to treat other types of pain as well. Always massage abdominal area in a clockwise motion.

- **To alleviate fatigue:** add 2 drops of thyme essential oil to your bath water diluted in almond, coconut, or rice milk.

- **For improved and restful sleep:** add a few drops to your diffuser.

- **To reduce the appearance of scars and skin marks:** apply thyme essential oil mixed with any carrier oil (like almond oil) on the affected area.

- **For use as a facial and skin cleanser:** mix a few drops of thyme essential oil into your facial wash product.

- **Use as a treatment or to protect against respiratory problems:** add 2 drops of thyme essential oil to hot water and use for steam inhalation.

- To uplift a sad mood, add 2 drops to a dampened cloth, cotton ball, or handkerchief and inhale the revitalizing scent of thyme essential oil.

Cautions

Thyme essential oil should not be used directly on skin as it can cause allergic reaction.[111] Dilute with a carrier oil like olive oil or almond oil. Before use, be sure to do a skin test.

Thyme essential oil is not recommended for people with hyperthyroidism because it may overstimulate the thyroid gland.[112]

Thyme essential oil can increase circulation; therefore people with high blood pressure should avoid it. Pregnant women should avoid thyme essential oil because it can

---

111   "Thyme Oil," www.healthy-holistic-living.com/thyme-oil-natural-antibiotic.html.

112   Joseph Mercola MD, "Thyme Oil," articles.mercola.com/herbal-oils/thyme-oil.aspx.

stimulate menstrual flow. Due to its strength, thyme essential oil should not be used on infants and young children.

Blends Well With

Lavender, lemon, orange, and rosemary essential oils.

Supernatural Uses

- Drops of thyme essential oil on a 1" piece of cloth can attract good health.

- Use drops of thyme essential oil for healing spells.

- A few drops of thyme essential oil placed on a cloth beneath a pillow bring restful sleep without nightmares.

- A magical, cleansing bath of marjoram and thyme essential oil drops removes past sorrows and ills.

- Drops of thyme essential oil worn on clothing allow the wearer to see fairies.

- A drop of thyme essential oil on clothing will also give the wearer courage.

- Sniffed, thyme essential oil, will bring courage and energy to any situation. Use a drop or two on a cotton ball and sniff gently.

- Diffused, thyme essential oil will purify your space.

12: Ylang-Ylang

Ylang-ylang is the Malay name for "flower of flowers." It comes from a small tropical tree native to the Philippines. Cultivated trees provide the floral, heady, sweet aroma of ylang-ylang whereas wild ones do not provide the same desirable, intense scent. In Asia, the flowers have long been valued for their aphrodisiac fragrance, originally extracted by maceration in coconut oil.

Its name originates from:

Latin: *Cananga odorata*	**French:** *Ylang-ylang*
Spanish: *Ylang-ylang*	**English:** *Ylang-ylang*
Gender: *Feminine*	**Ruling Planet:** *Venus*
Element: *Earth/Air*	

Property Description

Antidepressant, aphrodisiac, antiseptic, antispasmodic, anti-inflammatory, antiparasitic.

Benefits

Emotional clearing, insomnia relief, dispels negativity, alleviates jealousy, reduces anger, and lowers fever. Combats low self-esteem and restores confidence. Also known for its ability to help regulate cardiac arrhythmia, forestall hair loss, and neutralize intestinal problems.[113]

French chemists Garnier and Rechler recognized ylang-ylang's medicinal properties at the beginning of the twentieth century during their research on Reunion Island where they found ylang-ylang to be effective against malaria, typhus, and infections of the intestinal tract as well as have a calming effect on the heart.[114]

Ylang-ylang essential oil is primarily used for its positive psychological properties and helping people to overcome negativity, fears, inhibitions, feelings of low self-worth, self-hatred, inferiority, and insecurity.

Ylang-ylang essential oil is used for soothing insect stings and bites as well as general skincare.

It is steeped in coconut oil to produce a fragrant pomade called *boori-boori* which is used as a body rub to prevent fever and infections as well as nourish and rejuvenate the skin.[115]

---

113   Josh Axe, "Ylang-Ylang Boosts Heart Health, Moods & Energy," draxe.com/ylang-ylang/.

114   materiaaromatica.com,

115   www.junoskincare.com/#!ingredients/.

Background

Sometimes called "cheap man's jasmine," "crown of the east," or "perfume tree," ylang-ylang is visible along the roadside throughout Malaysia where it is planted on purpose to provide shade by day and a beautiful scent in the night air.[116] It is also used for decoration at festivals and celebrations combined with jasmine, rose, and champaca.[117]

Ylang-ylang essential oil is often used as an ingredient for aphrodisiac incense blends. In Southeast Asia, the flowers are spread on the wedding bed for extra special sensuous arousal because the scent is reputed to relax and calm wedding night fears and anxieties.

The Victorians added ylang-ylang essential oil in their Macassar hair oil products to encourage hair growth and bring a glossy sheen to their locks.[118]

Ylang-ylang essential oil assists in reuniting our emotional and sensual natures if they have wandered apart. It is a centering essential oil and unites the heart and the mind to soothe, open, and harmonize with the body.

COMMON USES FOR YLANG-YLANG ESSENTIAL OIL

- Diffused, ylang-ylang essential oil can be used to help chest infections, bronchitis, and spasmodic coughs.

- Ylang-ylang essential oil can be used on different types of skin—sensitive and oily as well as dry and mature due to its skin renewing and moisture retention properties. Add a few drops of ylang-ylang essential oil to your favorite body cream or facial tonic for softer and rejuvenated skin.

- Ylang-ylang essential oil is nourishing and moisturizing for dry, dehydrated, or irritated skin (see mix on next page):

---

116 www.cbd.int/cop/cop-11/doc/cop-11–commemoration-en.pdf.

117 "Ylang-Ylang," materiaaromatica.com/Default.aspx?go=Article&ArticleID=221 ;materiaaromatica.com/Default.aspx?go=Article&ArticleID=221.

118 Ibid.

Dry skin face cream:
Use 50 ml or 1.75 oz. of base cream or lotion. Add:
2 drops ylang-ylang essential oil
3 drops geranium essential oil
3 drops neroli essential oil
2 drops palma rosa essential oil
3 drops orange essential oil
Blend together.

- Ylang-ylang essential oil blends well with exotic essential oils such as vetiver and patchouli and can be used for its aphrodisiac properties in a romantic blend. Mix 2 drops of each for a diffuser or add the same mix of essential oils to ¼ C almond or jojoba oil for a delightful massage blend.

- Add several drops of ylang-ylang essential oil to your favorite shampoo or conditioner if you suffer from split ends.

- Make an overnight miracle moisturizing hair treatment using 4 to 6 drops of ylang-ylang essential oil mixed with 1 or 2 tsp. coconut or jojoba oil. Massage into hair, place a shower cap on your head and allow this to permeate your hair overnight.

- Combine 3 drops of ylang-ylang essential oil with 1 drop each of bergamot, sandalwood, vetiver, geranium, and lavender essential oils for a diffuser blend to relieve symptoms of menopause or the suffering of PMS. Massage pelvic area clockwise.

- Add a few drops of ylang-ylang essential oil to your bath for relaxation. Disperse in almond, coconut, or rice milk.

- For circulatory health, mix 2 to 3 drops of ylang-ylang essential oil in 1 oz. of carrier oil and massage on the body.

- Use for an upset stomach or mild food poisoning. Mix 2 to 3 drops of ylang-ylang essential oil in 1 oz. of carrier oil and gently massage on the stomach in a clockwise direction.

- To stimulate hair growth, mix 4 drops ylang-ylang essential oil with 1 T of carrier oil and massage into scalp. Leave on 20 minutes and shampoo out.

- For use as an aphrodisiac or to help alleviate frigidity or impotence, drop 8 to 10 drops of ylang-ylang essential oil in a bath using a dispersant like coconut, almond or rice milk. Soak for 20 to 30 minutes.

- To release anger or frustration, diffuse 1 drop ylang-ylang essential oil with 2 drops frankincense essential oil.

- For a really sexy night, diffuse 8 drops ylang-ylang essential oil with 6 drops sandalwood and 9 drops orange essential oils.

- For a calming and peaceful feeling, diffuse 3 drops ylang-ylang essential oil with 3 drops marjoram and 4 drops Roman chamomile essential oils.

- To promote healthy self-esteem, blend 2 drops ylang-ylang essential oil with 1 drop of Bergamot essential oil. Diffuse or use in a massage oil.

Cautions

Avoid in the first trimester of pregnancy.

Excessive use can cause headaches and nausea. Avoid using on inflamed skin or skin affected by dermatitis.

Blends Well With

Vetiver, patchouli, lavender, bergamot, rose, cinnamon, frankincense, benzoin, clove bud, and orange essential oils.

Supernatural Uses

Calming, uplifting, enthusiastic, joyous.

- Use a few drops of ylang-ylang essential oil for love spells and potions.

- Add a few drops of ylang-ylang essential oil to a piece of cloth and place under your pillow to attract a love interest.

- Add a few drops of ylang-ylang essential oil to a piece of cloth and place under your pillow for reducing fear or apprehension.

There you have it: the primary palette of essential oils. You now have a solid beginning with these initial twelve essential oils. I found it was helpful to familiarize myself with one oil at a time and begin experimenting when I gained knowledge about each one. The process unfolded organically when I allowed time to get to know their properties and powers.

At any given time in your life, you might find yourself with more emotional needs than physical, so begin by using them to heal your spirit. If you have more pressing physical needs, start alleviating them using essential oils. Healing the mind leads to healing the spirit, and that usually leads to healing the body.

Of course the healing process can start anywhere in the body and work itself into the mind and spirit. Since everything is connected each part of you will benefit from using essential oils. Eventually all will meld into one, and essential oils will serve as your conduit to healing as a package deal.

You have been guided to learn about essential oils and I am excited about your journey. It's a wonderful one and I wish you much success as a healing artist as you work with your first palette of essential oils for yourself and others.

In chapter eight we'll look at another twelve essential oils in the secondary palette that can give you even more versatility in blending your essential oils. The next twelve are ones you can add to your color palette and collection. Take your time. Work with your first twelve, see what wonderful blends you can create, and then gradually move into your second set. There's so much more to come.

EIGHT

The Secondary Palette: The Next Twelve Essential Oils 13–24

Once you have become familiar with the primary palette of twelve essential oils, you are ready to move onto the secondary palette of oils thirteen through twenty-four. I hope you have already found some blends that you enjoy and have enhanced your life each time you use them. Moving ahead on your journey with essential oils you may want to include these additional twelve in your expanding collection.

13: Patchouli

Patchouli *(Pogostemon cablin)* was named because of a native mint plant found in Madras which defined it as: *pachchai* (green) + *ilai* (leaf). Patchouli grows well in warm and tropical climates. A bit fussy, it thrives in hot weather but not direct sunlight. The seed-producing flowers are very fragrant and blossom in late fall.

Patchouli essential oil is a common ingredient in perfume and incense. The plant produces a conditioning oil and a heavy, pleasing, earthy scent. It was made famous in the 1960s as a favorite oil for the hippie generation because it masked many odors associated with street living.

Its name originates from:

Latin: *Pogostemon cablin*	**French:** *Huile de patchouli*
Spanish: *Pachuli*	**English:** *Patchouli, putcha-pat*
Gender: *Feminine*	**Ruling Planet:** *Saturn*
Element: *Earth*	

Property Description

Relaxant, digestive, anti-inflammatory, antifungal, antimicrobial, insecticidal.

Benefits

Lessens hypertension; improves IBS and skin conditions like eczema and acne; helps expel fluid retention. Also functions as an insect repellant, wound healer, snake bite remedy, and burn-out remedy.

Patchouli essential oil has been popular in Asia and India for centuries. It has beneficial effects on skin and scalp conditions and is helpful in healing wounds and reducing the signs of scarring.

It is considered an excellent remedy for insect and snake bites, and has been used as a fumigant. Because of its distinctive odor, patchouli essential oil is an antidepressant and mood lifter used to balance the body and stimulate a weakened immune system. It is said to bring into harmony the three principal forces at work within the body: the creative center, the heart center, and the transcendental wisdom center at the crown.[119]

Background

Patchouli grows naturally in southeast Asia. Its bushy plant is harvested several times a year.[120] The leaves are hand-picked, and allowed to partially dry in the shade and ferment for a few days before the oil is extracted via steam.

---

119   Misty Rae Cech, "Patchouli History and Uses," www.incensewarehouse.com/Patchoulis
-History-and-Use_ep_25–1.html.

120   "Patchouli's History and Use," www.incensewarehouse.com/Patchoulis-History-and-Use
_ep_25–1.html.

Patchouli essential oil is affordable because it is frequently harvested and easily processed. Patchouli is also one of the few essential oils that actually improves with age along with frankincense, cedarwood, sandalwood, and vetiver essential oils.

A properly aged patchouli oil, like a fine whiskey, is more desirable than a freshly bottled one. And also like a fine whiskey, patchouli essential oil may be an acquired taste for some.

Patchouli essential oil has a varied history and is a recognizable fragrance in the clothing business. Dry goods and cloth exported from India were doused with this warm, spicy scent, used mostly as a moth deterrent during shipping and sea travel.

The smell of patchouli became a measure of true "Oriental" fabric. European garment makers and knock-off artists scented their imitation products with patchouli to hoodwink buyers into thinking they were the real deal.

Patchouli essential oil is classified as a sensual oil and may help people integrate their feelings when they seem to be out of touch with their bodies because it relieves inhibitions and assists with impotence and the fear of sex.

Common Uses for Patchouli Essential Oil

- **For an uplifting blend:** use 3 drops patchouli essential oil and 1 drop rosemary essential oil. You can also place a few drops of this blend in an oil diffuser pendant necklace and wear it.

- Brighten your spirits by combining 2 drops lemon essential oil, 2 drops patchouli essential oil, and 1 drop bergamot essential oil. This will uplift your mood and bring you a sense of joy. Diffuse or wear this blend.

- For sensual encouragement, mix together 1 drop geranium essential oil, 1 drop patchouli essential oil, and 1 drop bergamot essential oil. Diffuse or blend with a carrier oil and use as a massage oil blend.

- Add few drops of patchouli essential oil to your favorite face cream or lotion to improve complexion and give skin a natural lift.

- Eczema can be helped when a few drops of patchouli essential oil is mixed into 1 tsp. carrier oil like apricot seed or virgin olive oil and rubbed on affected areas.

- As a natural emotional balancer, 3 to 4 drops of patchouli essential oil mixed with a carrier oil and used as a massage blend can help IBS when rubbed in a clockwise direction on the stomach and lower intestine area.

Blends Well With

Vetiver, rosemary, sandalwood, frankincense, bergamot, cedarwood, myrrh, rose, citrus, clary sage, lemongrass, geranium, and ginger essential oils.

Cautions

Check with your doctor before using patchouli essential oil if you are taking any blood-thinning or blood clotting medications. Patchouli essential oil may inhibit blood clotting and could have interactions with drugs.[121]

Supernatural Uses

Patchouli essential oil has a spicy, deep, earthy scent and is frequently used because of its connection to the rich earth. Civilizations have counted on it to bring prosperity and abundance to homes and families. The oil is used in ceremonies and prayers for those who need financial or other types of blessings in their lives.

- 1 drop of patchouli essential oil is often combined with 1 drop of sandalwood or rose essential oil to attract love. Use on a 1" piece of cloth and carry with you or place beneath your pillow at night.

- Moisten a cotton ball with 1 or 2 drops of patchouli essential oil. Simply close your eyes and visualize the cash rolling in as you and inhale the scent to activate your attraction of money.

- Diffuse a few drops of patchouli essential oil to attract a partner and to heighten lust.

- Diffused, patchouli essential oil seems to lower sexual inhibitions in women, and lowers anxiety in men, thus improving sexual enjoyment for both sexes.

---

121   Tisserand and Young, *Essential Oil Safety*, 382.

- Anoint an icon representing children with patchouli essential oil, place it in a location where you can see it every day, and children will manifest.

14: Rose

No single flower in history has seen more accolades and popularity than the rose. Sixty-million-year-old fossils of the rose have been discovered in Asia and thirty-five-million-year-old rose fossils have been found in Oregon and Montana.[122]

The oldest species of rose predates humankind, coming from central Asia some sixty million years ago during the Eocene epoch. The oldest existing rose is the *rose gallica* or *French rose*.[123]

There are two main sources of rose essential oil: the damask rose, *Rosa damascena*, comes from gardens in Bulgaria, Turkey, the Middle East, China, and Russia; and the cabbage rose, *Rosa centifolia*, which is farmed in France, Morocco, and Egypt. For our purposes we will use *Rosa damascena* as our choice for rose essential oil.

Its name originates from:

Latin: *Rosa damascena*	**French:** *Rosa de Damas*
Spanish: *Rosa de Damasco*	**English:** *Damask rose, rose of Castille, Mohammadi rose*
Gender: *Feminine*	
Element: *Water*	**Ruling Planet:** *Venus*

Property Description

Antidepressant, antiphlogistic, antiseptic, antispasmodic, antiviral, aphrodisiac, astringent, bactericidal, choleretic, cicatrisant, depurative, emenagogue, haemostatic, hepatic, laxative.

Benefits

Damask rose essential oil soothes and harmonizes the mind and helps with depression, anger, grief, fear, nervous tension, headaches, and stress. It also addresses sexuality,

---

122   "History of the Rose," www.herbs2000.com/flowers/r_history.htm.

123   Ibid.

self-nurturing, self-esteem, and dealing with emotional problems. It is a laxative, aphrodisiac, can increase sperm count, is beneficial to the liver and stomach, is a blood purifier, and promotes spiritual love.

It can repair broken capillaries, soothe inflammation as well as skin redness, and is useful for eczema and herpes.

Rose essential oil's greatest benefit is that it unites the physical with the spiritual, thus righting a lot of imbalances between the body, mind, and spirit.

Background

Avicenna, a tenth-century Persian physician and philosopher, chose the rose as his first plant to distill. His works in medicine, metaphysics, and philosophy influenced Thomas Aquinas and European monarchs. His rose distillery in Shiraz was operational until 1612.

During unstable times in Europe people were more fixated on personal survival than rose gardens. We are eternally beholden to the Benedictine monks who preserved roses used for medicinal purposes in their apothecary gardens.

Across the pond, Empress Josephine was very fond of roses and created a "rose renaissance" by growing more than 250 varieties in her gardens at Malmaison. Emperor Napoleon gathered rose bushes from the lands he conquered to bring back blooming souvenirs for his lady's garden. She even commissioned a court portrait painter, Pierre-Joseph Redouté, to paint her roses. His *Les Roses* work filled three volumes and was published after Josephine's death.[124]

Rose essential oil has been used throughout history in the ancient art of aromatherapy as a healing tonic and mood-elevating supplement. Rose petals are not very high in oil content: a rose blossom contains only about 0.02 percent essential oil; therefore, it requires sixty-thousand roses to produce just one ounce of oil, or ten thousand pounds of rose blossoms to produce one pound of oil.

As a result of the quantity of blossoms required for production, rose essential oil tends to be expensive. However, its price does not prevent it from being one of the most popular essential oils available.

---

124   Jerry Haynes, "Josephine and Malmaison," www.rose.org/wp-content/uploads/2012/01
      /Josephine-and-Malmaison-article-2.pdf.

There are mainly three sources of rose-types for rose essential oil. These are the oldest roses (the "parents" of many other varieties) and are highly valued for their fragrance and perfume.

The first is *R. gallica*, the most prolific of all roses. Originally from China, it is also known as the French rose, Provins rose, or Rose of Anatolia.

The second is *R. centifolia,* which came from Persia and is called the Provence rose or Rose of Ispahan. It is a direct descendent from *R. gallica*.

The third is *R. damascena*, the damask rose, which hails from Syria. It is very heavily scented and is the most desirable of all rose varieties due to its fragrance and is because it is the most popular in aromatherapy.[125]

Originally damask roses were grown in the Middle East, aptly named for the city of Damascus. Rose essential oil comes in two main types, rose absolute and rose otto. They are both used for the same purposes.

Rose otto is said to be the best type of rose essential oil for aromatherapy because it is extremely heady and you may find that you need to use much less in a blend with other essential oils and it seems to keep longer than rose absolute. The color of rose absolute tends to be a dark orange to red with an intense, pungent rose aroma. It is preferred by perfumers and said to be closer in fragrance to the flower than an otto. Only your experience with each of them will determine your preference.

COMMON USES FOR ROSE ESSENTIAL OIL

- **To help clear up acne:** dab 1 drop of pure diluted rose essential oil on blemishes three times a day. Make sure you use a sterile cotton swab; if the antimicrobial power is too much for you, dilute it slightly with a carrier oil.

- Diffuse rose essential oil to help poor circulation and heart problems such as arrhythmia and high blood pressure. It can also be diffused or inhaled to boost liver and gall bladder functions.

- Diffuse a few drops of rose essential oil for asthma relief, coughs, hay fever, digestive system disorders, and for liver congestion and nausea.

---

125 "A History of the Rose," www.herbs2000.com/flowers/r_history.htm.

- Diffuse rose essential oil for clearing, cleansing, and regulating female sex organs and hormones. It provides an overall toning effect on the uterus.

- Rose essential oil is good for dry, mature, and irritated skin. Add a few drops to your favorite cream or moisturizer along with a drop or two of sandalwood essential oil.

- Diffused or inhaled, rose essential oil provides a feeling of well-being and happiness; it also calms a nervous or anxious mind.

- Diffused, rose essential oil can ease allergies, asthma, baby blues, headaches, migraine, and nervous tension. The June 2012 issue of *Complementary Therapies in Clinical Practice* published a study using a group of twenty-eight postpartum women. After four weeks of essential oil (rose and lavender) therapy, the results were quite remarkable. Not only did the women experience a significant decrease in postnatal depression scores, they also reported marked improvement in general anxiety disorder![126]

- Diffused or inhaled, a few drops of rose essential oil can help fight depression, anger, and grief while dealing with emotional problems such as sadness and loss. It is a great tonic for matters of the heart.

- **To reduce skin redness, fight inflammations, and fix broken capillaries:** use a few drops of rose essential oil with 1 tsp. of a carrier oil and massage into skin.

Cautions

Rose essential oil is nontoxic, nonirritant, and nonsensitizing but should not be used during pregnancy without the proper supervision of a credentialed Aromatherapist. Tisserand and Young suggest a maximum dilution of .6 percent due to the fact the oil may contain methyleugenol.[127]

---

126 "The Effects of Clinical Aromatherapy for Anxiety and Depression in High Risk Postpartum Women—A Pilot Study," www.ctcpjournal.com/article/S1744–3881(12)00040–0/fulltext.

127 Tisserand and Young, *Essential Oil Safety*, 405.

Blends Well With

Bergamot, Roman chamomile, clary sage, geranium, lavender, lemon, patchouli, neroli, sandalwood, ylang-ylang, helichrysum, and vetiver essential oils.

Supernatural Uses

Rose essential oil is used to promote healing, love, luxury, contentment, protection, happiness, and unconditional love.

Rose essential oil unites the physical with the spiritual. It is said that when you inhale rose essential oil you inhale the love and kisses of angels.[128]

- For purposes of attracting and keeping love, apply a few drops of rose essential oil to note paper for sending love letters.

- For personal contentment, apply a few drops of rose essential oil onto a 1" piece of cloth and place beneath your pillow.

- Place 2 drops of diluted rose essential oil in your palms, rub together, and inhale for protection, healing, and self-confidence.

- Rose essential oil diffused in a magical setting will summon your deepest feelings.

15: Black Pepper

A flowering vine, pepper (*Piper nigrum*) is native to India and has been used in Indian cooking for more than four thousand years. The name comes from the Latin, but originated in Sanskrit as *pippali,* the name for elongated peppers.

"The ancient history of black pepper is often interlinked (and confused) with that of long pepper, the dried fruit of closely related *Piper longum*. The Romans knew of both and often referred to either as 'piper'. With the discovery of chili peppers in the New World, the popularity of long pepper entirely declined."[129]

---

128   Michele Duquet, "5 Amazing Things You May Not Know about Rose Essential Oil," michelesorganics.wordpress.com/tag/rose-essential-oil.

129   "Pepper," *Ancient History Encyclopedia*, ancient.eu /Pepper/.

Peppercorns, often referred to as "black gold," were used as a form of commodity exchange and were used for trade. Historically, all of the black pepper found in Europe, the Middle East, and North Africa traveled from India's Malabar region.

Its name originates from:

Latin: *Piper nigrum*	**French:** *Poivre noir*
Spanish: *Pimienta negra*	**English:** *Black pepper*
Gender: *Masculine*	**Ruling Planet:** *Mars*
Element: *Fire*	

Property Description
Analgesic, antiseptic, antispasmodic, antitoxic, antifungal, aphrodisiac, digestive, diuretic, febrifuge, laxative, rubefacient, tonic.

Benefits
Black pepper essential oil is used in the treatment of pain relief, particularly rheumatism and muscular aches, chills and fevers, flu, and colds. It increases circulation, combats exhaustion, and is a tonic for the spleen and aids digestion. It helps fight obesity, fungal infections, and aids in tobacco cessation and other addictions.

Black pepper essential oil not only warms the body but also re-energizes the system. It has a spicy, pungent aroma with a slightly sweet tolerable overtone.

Background
It was interesting to discover that black peppercorns were used extensively in Egyptian mummification. Archaeologists found black peppercorns packed into the nostrils of Rameses II, placed there as part of the mummification rituals after his death in 1213 BCE.[130]

Pliny the Elder's *Natural History* describes pepper prices in Rome around 77 CE:

---

130   "Spices All Over the World," www.jamalafoods.com/spices-all-over-the-world-iii/.

"Long pepper … is fifteen denarii per pound, white pepper is seven, and of black, four." Pliny also complains that "there is no year in which India does not drain the Roman Empire of fifty million sesterces." [131]

Like cinnamon and cloves, pepper is one of the oldest known spices, and as you read above, one of the most revered. It has been used in India since 2000 BCE, and was even used as a currency during the siege of Rome in 408 CE, where "peppercorn rents" meaning very low rent payments were commonly given to landlords. It is said that Attila the Hun demanded three-thousand pounds of pepper as a ransom for the city of Rome.[132] Pepper packs power on many levels.

In medieval times, pepper trade routes were controlled by Arab traders, although Italian city-states like Venice and Genoa monopolized shipping lanes once the spice landed on Mediterranean shores. Pepper was costly to ship, especially along the treacherous four-thousand-mile Silk Road. It was a desirable spice, and Italian traders could essentially set their own prices. Pepper earned the status as a luxury item in medieval Europe. The Dutch still use the phrase "pepper expensive" to refer to an item of prohibitive cost.[133]

Eventually, the rest of Europe tired of paying high Italian prices for pepper imports and decided to take matters into their own hands. Explorers were assigned the task of pepper acquisition on their voyages. Heading east, Christopher Columbus, Vasco de Gama, Sir Francis Drake, and other explorers sailed off into the waters of exploration for gold, pepper, spices, and land. On a return trip to the Mediterranean, Columbus had his men stock the holds of his ships with what he believed to be peppers he paid for. But when he arrived back in Spain he discovered that he had been duped and his ships were full of worthless chili peppers instead of the priceless peppercorns he thought he was transporting.

---

131   Pliny, *Natural History,* (New York: Penguin edition), chapter 12, 14.

132   "What Attila Reputedly Demanded 3,000 Pounds of as a Ransom for the City of Rome," www .globalclue.com/clue/What_Attila_reputedly_demanded_3000_pounds_of_as_a.

133   Stephanie Butler, "Off the Spice Rack: The History of Pepper," www.history.com/news /hungry-history/off-the-spice-rack-the-story-of-pepper.

Common Uses for Black Pepper Essential Oil

- **To relieve constipation:** mix 2 drops black pepper essential oil and 2 drops marjoram essential oil with 1 T of carrier oil for an abdominal clockwise massage.

- **To regulate the appetite:** diffuse a few drops of black pepper essential oil.

- Flatulence is relieved when a few drops of black pepper essential oil is inhaled or diffused.

- Use diluted black pepper essential oil in a compress to treat chilblains and bruises.

- **To cope with ongoing stress:** diffuse 3 drops black pepper essential oil and 3 drops orange essential oil.

- Diffused or inhaled black pepper essential oil will help fight addictions and encourage weight loss.

- **To warm cold feet:** soak them in a warm water basin with 2 drops black pepper essential oil disperse in coconut, almond, or rice milk.

- **For indigestion, gas and bloating, and to improve peristalsis:** mix 2 drops of black pepper essential oil with 2 drops peppermint essential oil and 1 drop Roman chamomile essential oil diluted in a carrier oil to make a stomach massage. Work clockwise.

- Diffused or inhaled, black pepper essential oil energizes and helps you move on when you feel stuck and trapped.

- Combine 1 to 2 drops of black pepper essential oil with 1 or 2 tsp. carrier oil to soothe sore muscles and joints or to warm the skin during wintery and rainy weather.

- Diffuse or inhale a few drops of black pepper essential oil to soothe anxious feelings.

- Diffuse or dilute 1 drop black pepper essential oil in 1 tsp. carrier oil and rub over the heart center as desired for emotional support.

- For extra energy, massage 1 or 2 drops of black pepper essential oil diluted in a carrier oil onto the soles of the feet daily, or diffuse as needed for increased energy.

- For a foot rub, add 5 drops peppermint, 3 drops clove bud, 5 drops Roman chamomile, and 3 drops black pepper essential oils with 2 T carrier oil placed in a 5–10 ml roller bottle.

- **To summon inner strength:** diffuse 2 drops basil essential oil, 2 drops bergamot essential oil, 1 drop cinnamon essential oil, 1 drop lemon essential oil, and 1 drop black pepper essential oil.

- **To promote circulation:** blend a few drops of black pepper essential oil into 1 T carrier oil or preferred lotion and apply to chest and limbs. Start at the center and work outward.

Cautions

Test the skin with a small amount of black pepper essential oil to check for sensitivity or possible allergic reaction.

Black pepper essential oil may cause irritation to sensitive skin; using too much could over-stimulate the kidneys.

It should be avoided in pregnancy and nursing due to its possible skin sensitizing effect. Avoid using in baths or massage if you have sensitive or allergy-prone skin. Avoid using if the oil has oxidized.[134]

Make sure you test-inhale black pepper essential oil before using it in case you are sensitive to the herb. (Do a sniff test by using a tiny amount of oil on a toothpick and gently inhale the scent to determine how you react to the essential oil.)

Blends Well With

Frankincense, lavender, marjoram, rosemary, cinnamon, sandalwood, clove bud, palo santo, ginger, and other spicy essential oils.

---

134   Tisserand and Young, *Essential Oil Safety*, 384–385.

Supernatural Uses

Fiery, stimulating, courage, bravery, fortifying, action-oriented.

Generates positive energy for change, enhances courage; protects against the evil eye and spells. Helps confront fears and can be used in exorcism rituals.

- 2 drops of black pepper essential oil dropped onto a cotton ball and inhaled dissolves spiritual exhaustion, and breaks through self-doubt.

- 1 drop diluted black pepper essential oil rubbed between palms and inhaled revives inner conviction and gives you strength to act.

- Diffused black pepper essential oil acts as a mild aphrodisiac.

- Curb unwanted addictions and obsessions by diffusing black pepper essential oil whenever you feel a pull to unwanted habits.

16: Clary Sage

The English name "clary" originates in the Latin *sclarea*, a word derived from *clarus* (clear). "Clary" was gradually modified into "clear eye," one of the popular names generally explained by the fact that the seeds have been employed for clearing the sight. The seeds are mucilaginous and a decoction from them placed in the eye would clear it from any small foreign body causing irritation. Regardless of the name, this essential oil is *not* to be used in your eyes.

Its name originates from:

Latin: *Salvia sclarea*	**French:** *Sauge sclarée*
Spanish: *Clary sage*	**English:** *Clary sage, clear eye, see bright, eyebright, clary, clary wort, muscatel sage*
Gender: *Feminine*	
Element: *Water*	**Ruling Planet:** *Moon*

Property Description

Antidepressant, anticonvulsive, antispasmodic, antiseptic, aphrodisiac, astringent, bactericidal, carminative, stimulant, deodorant, digestive, emenagogue, euphoric, hypotensive, nervine, sedative, stomachic, and uterine agent.

Benefits

Clary sage essential oil is used to enhance the immune system, calm digestive disorders, reduce inflammation from eczema, calm muscle spasms, and relieve respiratory ailments. It can help menstrual issues (cramps and hot flashes), promote relaxation during childbirth, and ease menopause symptoms.[135]

Herbalists in many regions of the world have traditionally used clary sage essential oil to ease the painful tightening of the uterus during childbirth. Clary sage essential oil is frequently combined with geranium essential oil to facilitate controlling as well as alleviating disorders endured by women from hormonal imbalances like menopausal symptoms, irregular menstrual periods, depression, headache, and nausea. For relief of feminine symptoms, use a cool towel compress of diluted clary sage essential oil. The use of a similar compress, warmed, is also helpful in alleviating liver, stomach, and gall bladder problems.[136]

Clary sage essential oil is used to calm the nervous system, especially during times of stress, depression, and insomnia. It can provide anxiety-lifting effects.

Background

Common clary, like garden sage, is native to Syria, Italy, southern France, and Switzerland, but will thrive in almost any soil that is not overly watered or continuously moist.

According to Michael Ettmueller, this herb was first brought into use by the wine merchants of Germany, who infused it with elder flowers, and then added the mixture to Rhenish wine, which converted it into a Muscatel. To this day in Germany it is still called *Muskateller Salbei*, Muscatel sage.[137]

---

135   "Clary Sage Oil, the Gentler Oil," articles.mercola.com/herbal-oils/clary-sage-oil.aspx.

136   "Aromatherapy Tip of the Day–Clary Sage," herbalriot.tumblr.com/post/56880555724 /aromatherapy-tip-of-the-day-clary-sage.

137   M. Grieve, "Clary Sage," www.botanical.com/botanical/mgmh/c/clacom72.html.

In other parts of the country, wine was made from the flowers of the herb. Combined with boiled sugar, it had a flavor like Frontiniac.[138]

In the Jura district of France, in Franche-Comte, the herb is supposed to mitigate mental and bodily grief, and Samuel Pepys in his *Diary* says:

> Between the cities of Gosport and Southampton (fourteen miles apart) we observed a little churchyard where it was customary to sow all the graves with sage. [139]

Clary sage is commonly known as "the gentler essential oil."

Common Uses for Clary Sage Essential Oil

- **To break up mucus in the lungs:** use 1 to 3 drops clary sage essential oil in a diffuser.

- **For relief of rheumatic pain and inflammation:** mix 3 drops of clary sage essential oil with 1 drop frankincense essential oil, 1 drop of eucalyptus essential oil, and 1 drop of yarrow essential oil, to 1 T of carrier oil and massage on inflamed or painful areas or joints.

- **For general pain relief:** mix 2 drops clary sage essential oil with 2 drops Peppermint essential oil and 3 drops lavender essential oil then mix with 1 T carrier oil and rub onto affected areas.

- Diffuse the above recipe (reducing carrier oil to 1 tsp.) when you need to see the big picture and get away from the minutia of the day.

- For a pick-me-up, mix 7 drops clary sage essential oil with 10 drops frankincense and 8 drops orange essential oil. Diffuse or mix with a carrier oil for a massage.

---

138   Sometimes with the words "white," "red," or "brown" appended, is an alternative and widely used name for muscat à petits grains. The term is often applied to table wines made from the variety; fortified wines use the abbreviated nomenclature of muscat.

139   M. Grieve. "Sages," www.botanical.com/botanical/mgmh/s/sages-05.html.

- **For emotional support:** mix 1 drop of clary sage essential oil with 1 drop each of sandalwood and lemon essential oils, diffuse.

- **Reward and refresh yourself:** inhale or diffuse 1 drop each of clary sage, lavender, and marjoram essential oils.

- **For hot flashes:** diffuse 1 drop clary sage essential oil with 1 drop basil, 1 drop lavender, and 1 drop rose essential oil.

- **For help with hair loss:** add a few drops of clary sage essential oil to your shampoo to stimulate hair growth. Clary sage essential oil can also alleviate dandruff.

- **To prevent infections:** Clary sage essential oil can be used to cleanse wounds and may help protect the body during surgery and against other infections. Mix 3 drops clary sage essential oil to 1 tsp. carrier oil. Apply carefully.

- **Diffused:** Clary sage essential oil can help relieve headaches, back pain, muscle stiffness, and cramps.

Cautions

Do not use clary sage essential oil during the first trimester of pregnancy. Do not use if you are consuming alcohol as it can cause hyper-intoxication.

Clary sage essential oil is generally a safe and nontoxic essential oil but may have some possibilities of irritating mucous membranes.[140] Inhale clary sage essential oil carefully and in small amounts to prevent excessive states of euphoria.

Note: Don't confuse clary sage essential oil with *Salvia officinalis* or common sage essential oil, which is not recommended due to the high content of thujone, a toxic substance.[141]

Salvia lavandulaefolla or Spanish sage essential oil has many aromatherapy uses but is not likely to offer the same benefits as clary sage essential oil either. They come from the same genus but have different properties.

---

140 "Clary Sage Essential Oil," www.auracacia.com/prdDisp.php?I=190811&full=y.

141 "Clary Sage," www.webmd.com/vitamins-supplements/ingredientmono-407–CLARY%20 SAGE.aspx?activeIngredientId=407&activeIngredientName=CLARY%20SAGE.

Blends Well With

Bergamot, frankincense, geranium, cedarwood, lavender, and sandalwood essential oils.

Supernatural Uses

Enhances dreaming; is protective, calming, balancing; brings in wisdom of the sages; lifts melancholy, paranoia, and stress.

- Sprinkle drops of clary sage essential oil around the table or surface on which you lay your tarot cards, runes, bones, or stones.

- Rub 2 drops of clary sage essential oil in your hands and inhale its fragrance to elicit inner wisdom.

- **For a personal aura cleanse:** mix 25 drops clary sage essential oil with ½ tsp. vodka in a 50 ml mist bottle filled with spring water. Spritz, don't drink! (Vodka helps disperse the oil and keep it mixed with the water.)

- Mix 2 drops clary sage essential oil with 1 C warm water to make an excellent clearing and enhancing wash for scrying mirrors and scrying stones.[142]

- Diffuse clary sage essential oil or anoint the third eye during any of these types of activities to enhance your visioning abilities and the reading.

- A drop or 2 of clary sage essential oil placed on a cloth or tissue under your pillow before bed can enhance any dream work and aid in the recall of dreams, especially for divination purposes.

- Clary sage essential oil enhances the ability to dream vividly. Mix 5 drops clary sage essential oil with 8 drops cedarwood essential oil and 12 drops thyme essential oil.

- **To connect with the universal energies:** mix 1 drop of clary sage essential oil with 1 drop each of myrrh and bergamot essential oils.

---

142   Scrying is an ancient technique for divination and telling the future.

17: Ginger

Zingiber officinale, a spice originally from the same family as cardamom and turmeric, ginger was discovered in the jungles of southern Asia.

Its early discoverers seasoned food and meats with the root and it has been used in international cuisines for centuries.

As a digestive aid, Confucius wrote as far back as 500 BCE of never being without ginger when he ate.[143] In the famous *De Materia Medica* written in 77 CE, Dioscorides recorded that ginger "warms and softens the stomach."[144] It also became popular in the Caribbean where the spice could be easily grown.

In the fifteenth century, ginger plants were transported by sea-going traders on ships destined for the Caribbean and Africa. Its popularity flourished; today ginger can thrive as a crop pretty much anywhere throughout the world.

Its name originates from:

Latin: *Zingiber officinale*	**French:** *Gigembre*
Spanish: *Jengibre*	**English:** *Ginger*
Gender: *Masculine*	**Ruling Planet:** *Mars*
Element: *Fire*	

Property Description
Anti-inflammatory, anticoagulant, digestive, expectorant, anesthetic, antifungal, stimulant.

Benefits
Reduces pain and inflammation; relieves arthritis, aching muscles, poor circulation, head-aches, and menstrual cramps. Its warming effect stimulates circulation.

---

143   Martha Whitney, "History of Ginger," herballegacy.com/Whitney_History.html.

144   J. W. Purseglove, E. G. Brown, C. L. Green, and S. R. J. Robbins, *Spices* vol. 2, (New York: Longman, 1981), 447–532.

It inhibits rhinovirus, common cold, bacteria like salmonella, inhibits diarrhea, protozoa, and Trichomonas.[145]

Reduces gas and painful spasms in the intestines and can help prevent stomach ulcers caused by the overuse of nonsteroidal anti-inflammatory drugs, such as aspirin and ibuprofen. Helps to alleviate respiratory infections and congestion. Aids indigestion, stomachaches, dyspepsia, colic, spasms, diarrhea, flatulence, and other stomach- and bowel-related problems.

Medicinally, ginger was reported to suppress human promyelocytic leukemia (HL)-60 cells.[146]

The most common and well-established use of ginger throughout history is probably its utilization in alleviating symptoms of nausea and vomiting.[147] Ginger has also been used for centuries in treating respiratory illnesses and is reported to contain potent compounds capable of suppressing allergic reactions.[148]

Another health claim attributed to ginger is its purported ability to decrease inflammation, swelling, and pain.[149] In addition to its effects in relation to cancer, some evidence supports a protective role for ginger in cardiovascular function and a number of other disease conditions.[150]

---

145 Linda Williams MD, "Benefits of Ginger," www.everydayhealth.com/columns/white-seeber -grogan-the-remedy-chicks/health-benefits-ginger.

146 S. O. Kim, K. S. Chun, J. K. Kundu, Y. J. Surh, "Inhibitory Effects of [6]-gingerol on PMA-induced COX-2 Expression and Activation of NF-kappaB and p38 MAPK in Mouse Skin." *Biofactors* 21(1–4), 2004: 27–31.

147 S. A. Boone and K. M. Shields, "Treating Pregnancy-Related Nausea and Vomiting with Ginger." *Annals of Pharmacotherapy* 39 (10), 2005: 1710–1713.

148 C. Y. Chen, Y. W. Li, S. Y. Kuo, "Effect of [10]-gingerol on [Ca2+]i and Cell Death in Human Colorectal Cancer Cells." *Molecules* 14(3), 2009: 959–969.

149 H. Y. Young, Y. L. Luo, H. Y. Cheng, W. C. Hsieh, J. C. Liao, W. H. Peng. "Analgesic and Anti-inflammatory Activities of [6]-gingerol." *Journal of Ethnopharmacology* 96 (1–2), 2005; 207–210; and P. Minghetti, S. Sosa, F. Cilurzo, et al, eds., "Evaluation of the Topical Anti-inflammatory Activity of Ginger Dry Extracts from Solutions and Plasters" *Planta Medica* 73 (15), 2007: 1525–1530.

150 R. Nicoll and M. Y. Henein, "Ginger (Zingiber officinale Roscoe): A Hot Remedy for Cardiovascular Disease?" *International Journal of Cardiology* 131 (3), 2009: 408–409.

The most common medical use of ginger is to alleviate the vomiting and nausea associated with pregnancy, chemotherapy, and some types of surgery. There is clinical data stating that ginger is at least as effective, and may be better, than vitamin B6 in treating these symptoms. Ginger also appears to reduce cholesterol and improve lipid metabolism, thereby helping to decrease the risk of cardiovascular disease and diabetes.[151]

Background

Ginger as a spice goes back five thousand years to the Vedic Indians and the ancient Chinese who believed it to be a tonic and the universal root for all ailments. The ancient Hindu epic poem, *Mahabharata,* referred to ginger as one of the spices used to cook meat.[152]

It was used extensively by the spice-loving Romans who imported it from India. When Roman rule was crushed, the Arabs cleverly seized control of the spice trade and all spices skyrocketed in price. The most popular were black pepper and ginger. In thirteenth-century Europe a pound of ginger was valued as the price of one live sheep.

Ginger has been a trading commodity as long as any other herb or spice. It came into its glory during the thirteenth and fourteenth centuries. Arab sailors wisely planted the rhizomes in Africa and Zanzibar thus spreading the cultivation of this great herb and making it more readily available.

In the sixteenth century Henry VIII was recommending it as remedy for the plague while his daughter, Queen Elizabeth, was in the kitchen inventing what now we call the gingerbread man.[153]

In 1852 an unfermented, nonalcoholic version of ginger beer was first made for children and nondrinkers by Dr. Cantrell in Belfast, Ireland, a well-known manufacturer of aerated and mineral waters. He called it "ginger ale" and the concoction tasted more intensely like ginger than the ginger-flavored beers of the day.[154]

---

151 Ann M. Bode and Zigang Dong, *Herbal Medicines: Biochemical and Clinical Aspects* second edition, via www.ncbi.nlm.nih.gov/books/NBK92775/.

152 "The History of the Ginger Plant," www.gardenguides.com/109595–history-ginger-plant .html.

153 qginger.com/history.html.

154 Ibid.

Ginger spice is a common food additive today; it can be found in grocery stores and purchased for a few dollars.

COMMON USES FOR GINGER ESSENTIAL OIL

- **To alleviate motion sickness:** place 2 drops of ginger essential oil on a cotton ball and sniff 2 hours before traveling.

- **Prevent jet lag:** mix 4 drops ginger essential oil with 8 drops lavender, 3 drops peppermint, and 6 drops grapefruit essential oils. Mix with 1 oz. carrier oil. Dab onto wrists and the inner part of your elbow three to four times a day. In addition you can mix this blend with water in a mister and disinfect your hotel room by spritzing the air.

- **For depression relief, mood swings, and mental stress or exhaustion:** diffuse a few drops of ginger essential oil.

- **To relieve male impotency:** rub 2 drops of diluted ginger essential oil on your palms and inhale. Since ginger essential oil is aphrodisiac in nature, it is effective in eliminating impotency and preventing premature ejaculation.[155]

- For rapid relief of abdominal upset, place 1–2 drops of ginger essential oil onto a cotton ball and inhale for 5 minutes. Rest and inhale for another 5 minutes.

- **For nausea:** diffuse 2–3 drops of ginger essential oil 30 minutes before surgery and 2 hours after surgery. Discuss the use of any essential oil with your surgeon or anesthesiologist before trying it.

- **To increase circulation:** mix 2–3 drops of ginger essential oil in 1oz. carrier oil and massage neck and back concentrating on the spine and nerve endings. Use strokes outward from the spine and down the limbs.

- To increase well-being, diffuse 2 drops of ginger essential oil and 2 drops of bergamot essential oil.

---

155   "Health Benefits of Ginger Root,"www.organicfacts.net/health-benefits/ginger-root-oil.html.

- **For overworked muscles and stress:** Mix 2 drops ginger essential oil in 1 T carrier oil and massage onto sore areas. Use a warm moist cloth on top as a soothing compress.

- **For additional stomach help:** (external massage) mix 4 drops ginger essential oil, 4 drops peppermint essential oil, 8 drops basil essential oil, and 4 drops of vetiver essential oil with a carrier oil of your choice and massage on abdomen in a clockwise motion.

- Create easier breathing by putting 3 drops of ginger essential oil and 3 drops of thyme essential oil in a diffuser.

- **Energy in a bottle:** mix into a roller ball 2 drops ginger essential oil, 2 drops of basil, and 1 drop peppermint essential oils in 1 tsp. carrier oil. Roll onto feet, wrists, and back of neck.

- **Restorative massage:** 12 drops of ginger essential oil and 8 drops of ylang-ylang essential oil with 4 drops of sweet orange essential oils in 4 oz. of a carrier oil and enjoy the rub.

- **Alleviate procrastination:** Mix together and diffuse 3 drops ginger essential oil, 3 drops grapefruit essential oil, 1 drop orange or lemon essential oil, 1 drop peppermint essential oil.

Cautions

Ginger essential oil is very potent and should therefore be used carefully and with properly trained supervision.

Some therapists recommend making a stomach tonic tea with a drop of ginger essential oil or peppermint essential oil.

Only try this under the direction of a certified Aromatherapist using organic, toxin-free essential oils.

If you are taking prescription blood thinners, have a bleeding disorder, or have gallbladder disease avoid medicinal doses of ginger.

Pregnant women should use caution using ginger essential oil as it can stimulate the uterus. Cardamom essential oil may work as a substitute for you.

Blends Well With

Lemon, cedarwood, lime, eucalyptus, frankincense, geranium, rosemary, sandalwood, patchouli, myrtle, bergamot, rosewood, neroli, orange and ylang-ylang essential oils.

Supernatural Uses

Love, money, success, power.

- Inhaling a drop of diluted ginger essential oil rubbed between your palms before performing spells or incantations increases your body heat and intensifies the power.

- Plant whole ginger roots to attract money and sprinkle with 1 to 2 drops of ginger essential oil added to water the roots.

- Use drops of ginger essential oil on a 1" piece of cloth to attract money. Keep in your wallet.

- Using ginger essential oil in love spells or under your pillow at night will attract romance.

18: Orange

Orange essential oil is sunny, radiant, and brings happiness and warmth to the nose and mind along with a sense of cheerfulness and joy. It makes you want to dance! The common and official names are derived from the Sanskrit *nagaranga* and the Arabic *naranj*.

Its name originates from:

Latin: *Citrus sinensis*	**English:** *Orange, bigarade orange, bitter orange, Seville orange, (sweet) Portugal orange, China orange*
Spanish: *Naranja*	
French: *Orange*	
Gender: *Masculine*	
Element: *Fire*	**Ruling Planet:** *Sun*

Property Description

Anti-inflammatory, antidepressant, antispasmodic, antiseptic, aphrodisiac, antitumoral, carminative, diuretic, tonic, sedative, and cholagogue.

Benefits

Orange essential oil is used in aromatherapy to create the feeling of safety, happiness, and warmth while calming nervous digestive problems. It creates cold and flu relief, rids the body of toxins and stimulates the lymphatic system, and it assists collagen formation in the layers of the skin. It helps with insomnia, brightens a dull complexion, acts as a diuretic, reduces wrinkles, and has the amazing ability to foster sleep at night. Orange essential oil can be used effectively on the immune system, for colds and flu, and to eliminate toxins from the body.[156]

Background

Sweet oranges were mentioned in Chinese literature as far back as 314 BCE. Ch'u Yuan, who in his first poem, called "Li Sao," mentioned many plants, trees, and fruits of that period (314 BCE.) This was contemporaneous with the first mention of citrus fruits in European literature by Theophrastus (*ca.* 372–287 BCE) also in 310 BCE.[157] The earth-shaped fruit is also mentioned in ancient Arabic writings. How they got to Europe is uncertain but we can logically assume trees or cuttings were transported via the busy Arab traders who brought good and spices to the continent in the eleventh century.

Orange fruit is a hybrid of pomelo (*Citrus maxima*) and mandarin (*Citrus reticulata*). It has genes that are 25 percent pomelo and 75 percent mandarin. Orange essential oil is extracted from the orange peel by cold-pressing.

Orange essential oil is one of the most difficult oils to preserve. It has a shelf life of about 6 to 12 months.[158] Although carefully stored in a cool area away from light, you may get more months of potency.

---

156   "Orange Oils," www.essentialoils.co.za/essential-oils/orange.htm.

157   John Webber Herbert, *History of the Citrus Industry*, revised by Walter Reuther and Harry W. Lawton via websites.lib.ucr.edu/agnic/webber/Vol1/Chapter1.htm.

158   "Orange Mid-season Essential Oil," www.naturesgardencandles.com/candlemaking-soap -supplies/item/essen-23/-orange-midseason-essential-oil.html.

In 1987 orange trees were designated as the most cultivated fruit tree in the world. Orange trees are widely grown in tropical and subtropical climates for their sweet fruit. Statistics reported in 2013 from the United Nations Food and Agricultural Organization show that sweet oranges accounted for approximately 70 percent of all citrus production worldwide.

The fruit of the *Citrus sinensis* is considered a sweet, edible orange, whereas the fruit of the *Citrus aurantium* is considered a bitter orange. The bitter orange and edible orange trees bear a great resemblance to each other, but their leaf stalks show a marked difference; the bitter orange broadens to the shape of a heart. The volatile oil of the bitter orange peel is known as oil of Bigarade, and sweet orange oil as oil of Portugal.

Historically, oranges have been associated with generosity and gratitude, and symbolized innocence and fertility.[159] On Chinese New Year oranges are given as gifts to symbolize happiness and prosperity.

COMMON USES FOR ORANGE ESSENTIAL OIL

- Use 3 to 4 drops orange essential oil in a diffuser to help children and adults fall asleep at night and to alleviate the symptoms of cold and flu, nervous tension, and stress. Do not leave children unattended with the diffuser for more than a few minutes.

- **Flu, colds, and tension bath:** blend a few drops of orange essential oil with 1 tsp. of carrier oil and add to a warm bath for help easing cold and flu symptoms.

- Add 5 drops of orange essential oil to 1 oz. cream to clarify skin. (This becomes a phototoxic cream. Avoid the sun for 12 to 24 hours after application.)

- Orange essential oil supports collagen formation in mature skin. Add a few drops to 1 tsp. of carrier oil and massage onto face and neck or area of concern. (This blend is phototoxic, so only use when you are not going out in the sun for 12 to 24 hours.)

---

159 "Essential Oil Spotlight: Orange," challengetochangeinc.com/essential-oil-spotlight-orange/.

- **To lift your mood or relieve chronic anxiety:** diffuse 3 drops of orange essential oil for 30 minutes three times a day.

- **For depression:** Put 2 drops of orange essential oil on a cotton ball and inhale four times a day.

- **To relieve anxiety in children:** diffuse 3 drops in a diffuser no more than 3 minutes at a time, (keep diffuser twenty feet from the child), three times a day to reduce symptoms.

- Diffuse orange essential oil to flush the body of toxins, gas, and bloating and to help your body shed weight.

- **For energy:** make an inhaler with 2 drops lavender essential oil, 1 drop of ginger essential oil, and 3 drops of orange essential oil. Use the inhaler five times a day.

- Orange essential oil can be used as a slug deterrent in your garden. Mix a few drops of orange essential oil in a spray bottle with 1 C of water and spray plants to repel slugs.[160] Shake well before use.

- **Digestive problems:** Orange essential oil can be very helpful for IBS and other digestive issues. Mix 2 to 3 drops in 1 oz. of carrier oil such as olive or jojoba oil and massage on lower back and abdomen in a clockwise direction.

- **To control acne breakouts:** moisten a cotton ball and add 2 drops of diluted orange essential oil. Dab lightly on acne and blemishes to remove excess facial oils.

- For joint and muscle pain, use 2 to 3 drops mixed in 1 tsp. carrier oil and massage on affected area. (Can also be used with a hot compress.)

---

160   Kimber Watson, "How to Make Natural Garden Pesticides," www.apartmenttherapy.com /how-to-make-natural-garden-pesticides-169168.

- **To reduce skin inflammation associated with eczema and psoriasis:** use 2 to 3 drops in a carrier oil such as olive oil, jojoba, or sweet almond and massage on affected area.

- **Relieve gingivitis and mouth ulcers:** place 2 to 3 drops orange essential oil in a glass, add water, and mix. Swish around in your mouth to cover the area but do not swallow. Repeat as often as needed.

Cautions

Orange essential oil is phototoxic and makes your skin sensitive to the sun. After you apply orange essential oil, wait 12 to 24 hours before you go out in the sun. Be sure to follow up by using a SPF 50 sunscreen or better for protection. Sunscreen does contain chemicals, so choose the ones with the least harmful ingredients.

Blends Well With

Basil, black pepper, cinnamon, clove bud, ginger, eucalyptus, ginger, grapefruit, lavender, frankincense, sandalwood, ylang-ylang, and vetiver essential oils.

Supernatural Uses

Love fruit, divination, luck, money.

- A few drops of orange essential oil placed on the flowers of a wedding bouquet leads to wedded bliss.

- The Chinese believe orange essential oil brings good luck and fortune. Drops of the oil on money or coins will bring prosperity.

- Diffused, orange essential oil will draw abundance to the home.

- Place a few drops of orange essential oil above your doorway to welcome luck and money.

19: Helichrysum

Helichrysum is Greek for "gold of the sun": *helios* means sun and *chrysos* means gold.

Aromatherapy literature is full of praise and testimonials for this oil. This essential oil leaves a big impression with its delicacy and powerful efficacy.

It has the ability to heal skin tissue steadily and that quality alone incites a great demand for this essential oil. It's unlikely you will find a better wound healer and anti-aging agent than this one.

Also called immortelle, it is is a flowering plant from the daisy family. Its leaves have a strong aromatic smell and when crushed, release a distinct curry-like aroma.

It is a charming plant to have in a garden for the aroma of curry alone and its pure beauty. The flowering plant was also nicknamed *Immortelle* and *Everlasting* because it retains its lovely yellow color even after drying

Its name originates from:

Latin: *Helichrysum italicum*	**French:** *Helichrysum*
Spanish: *Helichrysum*	**English:** *Helichrysum,*
Gender: *Masculine*	*Everlasting flower, immortelle,*
Element: *Fire*	*strawflower, curry plant*
	Ruling Planet: *Sun*

Property Description
Antiallergenic, antitussive, astringent, cholagogue, cicatrizant, diuretic, expectorant, fungicidal, hepatic.

Benefits
Helichrysum is used to reduce inflammation, promote healing wounds and minor burns, stimulate digestion, promote detox, boost the immune system, heal scars, reverse the signs of aging in the skin, and fight fungal infections. It has been used to treat acne, anxiety, arthritis, cough, eczema, insect bites, and sunburn.

Background
Helichrysum oil has been dubbed "the super arnica of aromatherapy" for its remarkable ability to speed the healing of wounds, bruises, scar tissue, and even broken bones. [161]

---

161 "Helichrysum Essential Oil," www.starchild.co.uk/products/6564_3383_helichrysum
-essential-oil.aspx.

Helichrysum is most recognized for its effective skin treatment and in helping lung issues like congestion, allergies, and respiratory illnesses.

Helichrysum's tremendous regenerative properties are familiar to sprains, strains, sore tendons, muscle aches, and bruises. It has been studied in Europe for its healing effects on certain skin ailments, scar reduction, nerve regeneration, and inflammation.

Most notably in France, helichrysum has been marketed as an antiaging miracle oil and has been labeled as a fountain of youth in a bottle.[162]

There are more than five-hundred different species of helichrysum in the world today. There is only one used therapeutically, *Helichrysum italicum*. The best is produced in Corsica, a small Mediterranean island off the coast of France. Because it has properties that are very effective, you need to beware of imposters.[163]

Production of helichrysum essential oil is extremely limited on the small island, which counts just five distillers among its population of three hundred thousand. Julie Dawn, Helichrysum italicum expert, says:

It is so special because it treats cosmetic as well as medical problems. It can treat age spots to sports injuries. Known for its antibacterial qualities and its tissue healing properties, tests have been carried out at the hospital in Grasse, France, where they used *Helichrysum italicum* essential oil to close skin tissue. The result has been absolutely amazing as a very quick heal, very little scarring, no redness, and no infections. It multiplies the natural collagen count present in our skin cells and diminishes wrinkles and creases with a high percentage of success. It is also combined with other oils and used to treat acne.

Helichrysum essential oil acts on the skin, on muscles and joints, and on the nervous system; there are not many essential oils with this vast healing power. In fact I now call *Helichrysum italicum* "liquid gold," as it is so precious."[164]

---

162 "Helichrysum," veriditasbotanicals.com/how-to-use-our-essential-oils-therapeutically /helichrysum/.

163 "Helichrysum," veriditasbotanicals.com/how-to-use-our-essential-oils-therapeutically /helichrysum/.

164 Julie Dawn, "Helichrysum Essential Oil," www.helichrysum-italicum.com/helichrysum -oil-10–c.asp.

USDA researchers at Tufts University have developed a laboratory test to measure the oxygen radical absorption capacity of different foods and natural substances. Known as the ORAC scale, it is one of the most sensitive and reliable methods for measuring antioxidant capacity. Scoring in the top percentile, helichrysum essential oil provides a solid defense against harmful free radicals.[165]

COMMON USES FOR HELICHRYSUM ESSENTIAL OIL

- **Scar relief:** mix 2 drops lavender essential oil with 1 drop rosemary essential oil and 1 drop helichrysum essential oil in a carrier oil and apply to scars. Apply three to four times daily for fresh scars and up to 4 months for older scars. If you gently tap on the scar tissue with your fingers after applying the oils, you will find they heal faster.

- **For pain relief:** mix 5 drops of helichrysum essential oil with 10 drops of peppermint essential oil in 1 T carrier oil for an excellent general analgesic that relieves neck/back pain, TMJ symptoms, arthritis pain, and even restless leg syndrome. Allow the essential oil blend to penetrate skin for a couple of minutes. Repeat every 5 minutes until pain subsides.

- **Minor burn therapy:** apply undiluted as soon as possible for immediate relief. Use 1 to 3 drops of both helichrysum essential oil and Lavender essential oil mixed with 5 drops of a pure carrier oil as necessary.

- **Inflammation reducer:** for impact-type injuries you can apply undiluted immediately on the injury to prevent initial swelling and reduce healing time. Mix 10 drops helichrysum essential oil with 5 drops of German chamomile for further anti-inflammatory effects. Same formula applies for sprains and ankle twists. Repeat application every 30 minutes until you see and feel results.

---

165 "Helichrysum: Treat and Repair," www.helichrysum-italicum.com/index.html.

- **Another option for healing a scar:** use 1 drop of helichrysum essential oil with 3 drops lavender essential oil diluted in a carrier oil on any scar, new or old. Cover the entire scar area, tap gently on the scar tissue, and massage lightly to discourage development of scar tissue.

- **For tinnitus relief:** apply 1 drop diluted behind the ear. Apply a second drop to a cotton ball and place cotton in the ear while sleeping each night. This may take time to work.

- **For faster healing of cuts, wounds, and bruises:** use helichrysum essential oil topically, diluted.

- Use helichrysum essential oil topically to diminish stretch marks. Mix with a carrier oil and massage into marked skin.

- Helichrysum essential oil is also effective for sun-damaged skin. Dilute 2 drops of helichrysum essential oil in 9 drops of carrier oil and massage into skin.

- Diffused, helichrysum essential oil has strong purification properties and can be used to assist with detoxifying from the use of drugs or nicotine products.

- **For aging skin:** mix 5 drops of helichrysum essential oil with 3 drops frankincense, 2 drops of rose or sandalwood, and 3 drops of geranium essential oils, and mix half-and-half with carrot seed essential oil and pomegranate essential oil. Apply to face or add into a face cream (equal parts). Apply day and night for effective wrinkle relief.

Cautions
Avoid using during pregnancy.

Blends Well With
Bergamot, Roman chamomile, sandalwood, palo santo, ginger, grapefruit, geranium, lemon, orange, rose, and vetiver essential oils.

Supernatural Uses

Awareness, calm, patience, creativity, intuition, courage, endurance.

Heals physical and emotional scarring, opens the heart, connects body and spirit, and opens human beings to the spiritual part of their life. Helichrysum essential oil is one of the angelic fragrances.

- Rub 2 drops in the palms of your hands and inhale helichrysum essential oil to calm painful emotions.

- Diffuse helichrysum essential oil to encourage patience while trying to understand a difficult person or situation.

- Diffuse helichrysum essential oil for full awareness of the dangers and pitfalls of life.

- Use 3 to 5 drops in an aroma lamp or diffuser in your workplace to ignite creativity.

- **To stimulate intuition:** mix 8 to 10 drops in your bath and/or wear a couple of drops as a body perfume.

- Use a few drops in your diffuser of helichrysum essential oil for scrying and channeling rituals.

20: Vetiver

Vetiver (*Vetiveria zizanioides*) is a tall, tufted, scented grass with long narrow leaves native to India, Indonesia, Philippines, Tahiti, Java, and Haiti. It is botanically related to lemongrass and citronella. Vetiver essential oil is also known as the *oil of tranquility* because of its calming properties.

Vetiver grass was originally used in Calcutta and Haiti for thatching, awnings, blinds, and sunshades. In Java the roots were used for weaving mats and thatching huts. The fragrance of the vetiver plant not only gave rooms an exquisite fragrance but also deterred insects. Among its many attributes, the grass crop also protects against soil erosion while it grows.

Its name originates from:

Latin: *Vetiveria zizanioides*	**French:** *Vetiver*
Spanish: *Vetiver*	**English:** *Vetiver, khas-khas, khus-khus, khus grass, cuscus grass, moras*
Gender: *Feminine*	
Element: *Earth*	**Ruling Planet:** *Venus*

Property Description

Anti-inflammatory, antiseptic, antispasmodic, relaxant, circulatory stimulant, vulnerary, sedative.

Benefits

Helps with ADHD, anxiety, anger control, rheumatism, arthritis, depression, postpartum depression, insomnia, and skin care, especially wrinkles. As well as having a positive effect on hormonal imbalance and insomnia relief, vetiver essential oil has a calming and soothing effect on the nervous system and is helpful for muscular aches and pains.

Vetiver essential oil is deeply grounding and reputed to be an immunostimulant; effectively increasing and enabling the body's ability to withstand stress while strengthening the immune system. Vetiver essential oil is a core stabilizer and return us to the roots of earth's nurturing, healing energies.

This oil is highly recommended for those who are experiencing shock or traumatic events such as bereavement, divorce, or separation.

Vetiver essential oil also benefits people with rheumatism, arthritis, gout, muscular aches, and dryness and cracking of the skin.[166] Its scent reminds us of myrrh and patchouli. When it is diluted, its lemony overtones become more pronounced.

Vetiver essential oil is deeply relaxing, so it is extremely valuable in massage and baths for those experiencing stress be it chronic or temporary.

---

166 "Vetiver," www.botanicalsbythesea.com/store/p117/Vetiver_10_ml.html.

Background

Vetiver essential oil processing was introduced to Haiti in the 1940s by Lucien Ganot. Total production increased in ten years from twenty to sixty tons annually, making Haiti the largest producer in the world.[167]

Khus essence is a thick, dark green syrup made from the roots of khus (vetiver) grass. It has a woody taste and a scent characteristic of grass. Vetiver essential oil, as khus, is also used as a flavoring agent syrup. Khus syrup is made by adding khus essence to sugar, water, and citric acid syrup. The syrup is used to flavor milkshakes and yogurt drinks like lassi and can also be used in ice creams, mixed beverages like Shirley Temples, and as a dessert topping.[168]

COMMON USES FOR VETIVER ESSENTIAL OIL

- **For nervousness:** diffuse 2 or 3 drops vetiver essential oil to calm jangled nerves, dispel hysteria, anger, and irritability; and also to relieve insomnia.

- **Dry skin relief and moisturizer:** 5 to 10 drops of vetiver essential oil can be blended into 1 oz. of face cream or lotion to nourish the skin and is specifically beneficial to dry, irritated, and dehydrated skin.

- **Wrinkles and skin tone:** Vetiver essential oil is helpful in reducing wrinkles and stretch marks and to improve the tone of sagging skin, as well as helping wounds to heal. Mix with equal amounts of lavender essential oil and frankincense essential oil in a carrier oil such as apricot seed or pomegranate for beautiful skin renewal.

- **Muscle ache relief:** Combine 5 drops of vetiver essential oil, 3 drops of lavender essential oil, and 2 drops of eucalyptus essential oil with 1 T of carrier oil and rub into sore muscles. Reapply every 30 minutes until you feel relief.

---

167   "Khuskhus," www.gutenberg.us/articles/Khuskhus.

168   "Khus Syrup Glossary," tarladalal.com.

- **Moth repellant:** Soak a few cotton balls in a few drops of vetiver essential oil and place in your drawers and closets to protect clothes and linens.

- To help mature skin restore elasticity and tone, blend 5 drops of vetiver essential oil into 1 tsp. of organic face cream. Gently massage in an upward motion onto face twice daily.

- **Relieve insomnia:** prepare a bath with 2 drops vetiver essential oil, 4 drops sandalwood essential oil, and 1 T carrier oil. Soak for 20–30 minutes. You can also diffuse this same blend.

- **To suppress acne:** Vetiver essential oil can be effective in treating acne and dry skin. Use neat on eruptions. Blend with a carrier oil and 1 drop of lemon for a stronger face blend applied to a limited area. (Use at nighttime to avoid sun exposure for 12–24 hours.)

- **For stiff joints and rheumatism relief:** mix 2 drops vetiver essential oil with 4 drops ginger essential oil and 1 C Epsom salts. Allow essential oils to dissolve into the Epsom salts and add to a warm/hot bath right before you get in. Soak for 20 to 30 minutes.

- **Mental exhaustion relief:** mix 2 drops vetiver essential oil, 4 drops neroli essential oil, 4 drops peppermint essential oil, and 1 T carrier oil. Massage onto your body. You can also diffuse this blend.

Cautions

Vetiver essential oil is safe, nonirritating, nonsensitizing, and a nontoxic substance.

The best idea is to test inhale the vetiver essential oil scent and see how it makes you feel before going too gung-ho with it.

Tisserand and Young recommend a dermal maximum of 15 percent.[169]

Blends Well With

Pink grapefruit, ylang-ylang, sandalwood, patchouli, orange, helichrysum, geranium, lavender, clary sage, and neroli essential oils.

---

169   Tisserand and Young, *Essential Oil Safety.*

Supernatural Uses

Love, luck, money, spell-breaking, theft prevention. Psychologically grounding, vetiver essential oil helps cope with stress and recovery from emotional trauma.

- Place a few drops of vetiver essential oil on the cash register or money box to prevent theft.

- Inhale 2 drops vetiver essential oil rubbed on the palms of your hands to create a love attraction.

- Diffuse a few drops of vetiver essential oil and use positive affirmations to rid the room, person, or environment of evil spells or hexes.

- Diffuse a few drops of vetiver essential oil to help your heart with recovery from emotional trauma.

- Diffuse a few drops of vetiver essential oil in the room of a person suffering with ADHD.

- Diffuse vetiver essential oil to encourage patience when you need it. (Use one drop in diffuser for each person/situation that requires patience.)

21: Basil

Basil's history spans four thousand years, dating back to the first written accounts mentioning its cultivation in Egypt where it was possibly used in the embalming process.

At this stage, I'm thinking that most of our key essential oils were used for embalming by the wise Egyptians!

Basil *(Ocimum basilicum)* has two parts to its name and two meanings. Greek mythology suggests the origin of the first half of basil's scientific name came from the story of a warrior, Ocimus, who fought in Greece.

When Ocimus was felled by a challenging gladiator, the herb basil appeared.[170]

The second half of the scientific name for basil is derived from Greek word *basileus,* meaning "king" or "kingly." It has convincingly royal overtones.

---

170   "Basil," www.ourherbgarden.com/herb-history/basil.html.

Its name originates from:

Latin: *Ocimum basilicum*

Spanish: *Basilio*

Gender: *Masculine*

Element: *Fire*

French: *Basile*

English: *Basil, our herb, sweet basil, witches herb, albahaca, American dittany, St Joseph's wort*

Ruling Planet: *Mars*

Property Description

Analgesic, antidepressant, anti-inflammatory, antiseptic, antispasmodic, antiviral, decongestant, expectorant, and stimulant.

Benefits

Skin care, indigestion, respiratory problems, infections, stress disorders, blood circulation, pain, diarrhea, cough, mucous discharges, constipation, indigestion, some skin diseases, and vomiting.

Possessing anti-bacterial properties, basil essential oil is good for treating a variety of infections such as cuts, wounds, skin infections, bladder infections, and viral infections that enter the body through other cuts and wounds.[171]

Because of its refreshing effect when smelled or consumed, basil essential oil is used for treating nervous tension, mental fatigue, melancholy, migraines, and depression.

Basil essential oil is often used in the treatment of arthritis, wounds, injuries, burns, bruises, scars, sports injuries, surgical recovery, sprains, and headaches because it is an analgesic and provides relief from pain.

Background

Historically, basil was thought to be harmful. In ancient Greece and Rome, basil was feared and associated with poverty, hate, misfortune, and the devil because it was widely believed that basil could only prosper where abuse was present.[172] In fact, ancient Greek farmers are

---

171   "15 Health Benefits of Basil (Tulsi)," www.wellnessgyan.com/wellness/15–health-benefits-of -basil-tulsi-2232715.

172   "Basil," www.ourherbgarden.com/herb-history/basil.html.

alleged to have shouted and cursed when they planted basil seeds. After hearing them, the French coined the phrase: *semer le basilica*, a phrase referring to slander.[173]

Basil was given to young women to hold before marriage. If it withered, they were branded as unchaste. Along those same lines, basil was also thought to have transformative abilities. Lord Bacon in his *Natural History* wrote that basil, when exposed too much to the sun, would change into wild thyme.[174] These reactions were attributed as properties of the devil.

On the other hand, basil was considered to be a sacred herb in India. As such it was planted around temples for protection for the dead. Also called the Toolsee plant, basil was held as sacred by the Hindus and no offering to the gods could be complete without including holy basil leaves.

"Every good Hindu goes to his rest with a basil leaf on his breast. This is his passport to Paradise."[175]

Basil is native to Africa, India, and Asia. Some Greek Orthodox churches use it to prepare holy water. Pots of basil are set below church altars to honor the legend that basil was found growing around Christ's tomb. In India oaths were sworn upon it in courts because it was believe that basil contained a divine essence that imbued it with supernatural empowerments.[176] Such a complicated history for this lovely herb.

COMMON USES FOR BASIL ESSENTIAL OIL

- **To sharpen mental focus:** diffuse 3 drops lemon essential oil, 3 drops basil essential oil, and 2 drops rosemary essential oil.

- **To relieve fatigue:** massage 3 drops of basil essential oil diluted onto bottoms of feet mixed with 1 tsp. carrier oil.

- **Muscle soreness:** apply diluted basil essential oil directly on sore muscles.

---

173   "Basil," www.ourherbgarden.com/herb-history/basil.html..

174   "Basil," OurHerbGarden.com, http://www.ourherbgarden.com/herb-history/basil.html.

175   M. Grieve, "Basil, Sweet," www.botanical.com/botanical/mgmh/b/basswe18.html.

176   "Plant Finder," www.missouribotanicalgarden.org/PlantFinder/PlantFinderDetails.

- **Energy booster:** blend equal parts basil, peppermint, and grapefruit essential oils. Diffuse a few drops at a time.

- **Bathroom deodorizer:** mix equal parts basil, lavender, and lemon essential oils and place 2 drops of mixture in toilet water to keep the bathroom smelling fresh.

- **Freshen the air:** mix equal parts lemon, grapefruit, vetiver, and lavender essential oils together and diffuse.

- **For oily hair:** mix 1 drop basil essential oil with 2 drops lavender essential oil, 2 drops lemon essential oil, and 2 drops rosemary essential oil. Add 2 drops of the blend to a dollop of your shampoo. Leave on hair for 1 minute, then rinse.

- **Two refreshing and mood lifting basil essential oil blends:**
  1. In a diffuser use equal parts of basil, rosemary, peppermint, and orange essential oils.
  2. In a diffuser mix equal parts of basil and lemon essential oils.

- **To brighten and enhance skin:** massage a few drops of basil essential oil mixed into equal parts of a carrier oil into skin. Add a drop of lemon essential oil for extra brightening but don't go out in the sun for at least 12 to 24 hours if you add the lemon essential oil.

- **Relieve itchy skin:** mix 5 drops basil essential oil with 1 tsp. of carrier oil and massage onto itchy skin.

- **To curb nausea/motion sickness:** add one drop basil essential oil to a cotton ball and inhale for at least a minute. Repeat as needed.

Cautions

Basil essential oil and basil (St. Joseph's wort) in any other form should be avoided by pregnant, breastfeeding, or nursing women. Tisserand and Young recommend a dermal maximum of 15 percent if the level of eugenol is under .8 percent.[177]

177   Tisserand and Young, *Essential Oil Safety*, 208.

Blends Well With

Bergamot, cedarwood, geranium, helichrysum, lavender, lemon, lemongrass, rosemary, peppermint, and vetiver essential oils.

Supernatural Uses

Love, exorcism, wealth, flying protection, cheerfulness, integrity, trust, harmony.

- A few drops of basil essential oil, diluted, on the bodies of lovers fosters empathy between them. It soothes tempers and encourages peace.

- Massage a few drops of diluted basil essential oil over solar plexus and heart as needed for fear.

- Sprinkle a few drops of basil essential oil under your mattress to encourage fidelity.

- Place a few drops of basil essential oil onto paper currency and carry in your wallet to attract wealth.

- For fear of flying, cut a 1" piece of cloth and sprinkle basil essential oil on it. Carry close during air travel. The aroma will reduce fears.

- Add a few drops of basil essential oil to your garden water and use it to water your garden in order to protect your home.

- Coat an amulet with basil essential oil and carry it with you for success.

- Bring luck to a new home by gifting the owners with basil essential oil.

22: Neroli

It is not known precisely when or where neroli essential oil *(Citrus aurantium* var. *flos)* was first extracted but legend has it that during the seventeenth century in Italy, Anne Marie de la Trémoille (Orsini), duchess of Bracciano and princess of Nerola, first introduced neroli essential oil as a fashionable fragrance to high society. She used it in her bath and to perfume her stationery, scarves, and most famously, her gloves.[178]

---

178   Carmen Mychelin, "Orange Blossom: The Other White Flower," www.sniffapaloozamagazine .com/michorangeflowers.html.

Its name originates from:

Latin: *Citrus aurantium*	**French:** *Neroli*
Spanish: *Neroli*	**English:** *Neroli, orange flower oil, bitter orange flower*
Gender: *Masculine*	
Element: *Fire*	**Ruling Planet:** *Sun*

Property Description

Antiparasitic, digestive, antidepressive, hypotensive, bactericide, disinfectant, antispasmodic, emollient, sedative, tonic.

Benefits

Traditionally, neroli essential oil has been used to uplift mood and combat depression. Neroli essential oil is very relaxing and can relieve chronic anxiety, depression, fear, shock, stress, and insomnia. Its calming effect can also be beneficial to the digestive tract and can be effective for intestinal spasms, colitis, lowering blood pressure, and diarrhea.

Neroli essential oil stimulates cellular activity and helps to rejuvenate and regenerate the skin by increasing cell growth.[179]

Neroli essential oil is mostly used as an emotional remedy to help free mind and spirit of fears, and reinstate *joie de vivre*. It can even be used to help cases of hysteria, trauma, and shock.

Neroli essential oil helps insomnia and is one of the essential oils with the most sedative effects. It works to calm heart palpitations, headaches, neuralgia and vertigo. Neroli essential oil can help when a patient is convalescing and is a good general tonic.[180]

For the skin, neroli essential oil can help to regenerate skin cells and acts as a rejuvenating oil for scar tissue, stretch marks, and broken capillaries.

---

179 "Neroli Essential Oil," www.essentialoils.co.za/essential-oils/neroli.htm.

180 Ibid.

Background

It is believed that *Citrus aurantium* originated in southeast Asia, later spreading to northeastern India, Burma, and China, eventually finding its way via the Arab trade route to Africa and Syria. From these regions Moorish traders brought it to the Mediterranean, and by the end of the twelfth century it was grown and cultivated in Seville, Spain, where it was named for the city and given the common name for bitter oranges.

The fragrance of neroli essential oil caught on like wildfire in 1709 when the Italian perfumer J. M. Farina launched his blend of neroli, bergamot, lavender, lemon, petitgrain, and rosemary essential oils before an unsuspecting European continent, naming it *Eau de Cologne*.[181] That's a day to mark when this innovative industry opened a new world for the appreciation of scents.

Like rose and jasmine essential oils, neroli essential oil is a complete fragrance in and of itself. The oils produced in France and Tunisia have always been considered to be the very finest, commanding the highest price.

Much of the Tunisian neroli essential oil is produced from the blossoms of trees that are grown and farmed without agrochemicals and cultivated by co-operatives and families rather than high production commercial farms.[182]

The flowers of the bitter orange tree are the basis of neroli essential oil. The largest bitter orange tree plantations are in the south of France, in Calabria, and in Sicily. During the flowering season in May the flowers are gathered two or three times a week, after sunrise. After gathering, the flower buds and petals are immediately processed and distilled. There are two parts to the processing. The first is to appropriate the essential oil which rises to the surface and extract it. The second is for the leftover water, which is bottled and sold as orange flower water. Orange flower water is used in France, the Middle East, and England by bakers to give baked goods and pastries a crispy quality.[183]

In some Middle Eastern countries, drops of orange flower water are added to hard water drawn from wells to disguise the unpleasant taste. In the United States, orange flower water is used to make marshmallows.

---

181   "Johann Maria Farina," www.famousbirthdays.com/people/johann-farina.html.

182   "Essential Oils," 3wisemenessentials.com/essential_oils.html.

183   "Puddings, Custards and Creams" www.foodtimeline.org/foodpuddings.html.

Common Uses for Neroli Essential Oil

- **For energy:** diffuse 2 to 3 drops neroli essential oil.

- **For muscle spasms:** use 2 to 3 drops neroli essential oil in a diffuser or 4 to 5 drops blended into a carrier oil to improve colon problems, diarrhea, and nervous dyspepsia. Massage clockwise around middle torso area.

- **To alleviate anxiety, depression, hysteria, lethargy, panic, shock, or stress:** diffuse 3 to 4 drops neroli essential oil twice daily or add 4 to 5 drops diluted in coconut, almond, or rice milk to a warm bath.

- **For improved circulation:** mix 3 or 4 drops neroli essential oil in 1 oz. of carrier oil and massage on body stroking from the center outward.

- **For headaches and neuralgia:** place 3 to 4 drops in a warm or cold compress (whichever works best for you) and lay on forehead and neck.

- **For PMS:** diffuse 3–4 drops neroli essential oil or add 8 to 10 drops in bath water diluted in coconut, almond, or rice milk for a 20 minute soak.

- **Improve skin elasticity in mature skin:** mix a drop or 2 of neroli essential oil into 1 tsp. of unscented, natural face cream, and apply.

- **For irritability and sensitivity that can accompany menopause:** use 3 to 4 drops neroli essential oil in a diffuser or 8 to 10 drops in bath water diluted in coconut, almond, or rice milk, regularly. A body massage can also bring relief by mixing 3 to 4 drops in 1 oz. carrier oil and massage on body.

- **Diminish scars and stretch marks:** in 1 tsp. carrier oil dilute 3 to 4 drops neroli essential oil and 2 drops of helichrysum essential oil. Massage into affected areas.

- Diffuse a few drops of neroli essential oil for insomnia, vertigo, or depression, as well as anxiety and shock.

- **For stretch marks:** add 3 drops of neroli essential oil to a cream, lotion, or 1 tsp. of carrier oil and work into stretch marks or broken capillaries to activate scar healing.

Cautions

Neroli essential oil has calming and tranquilizing affects. Avoid using when driving a vehicle or operating other heavy machinery. Neroli essential oil is not considered phototoxic.[184]

Blends Well With

Benzoin, cedarwood, geranium, frankincense, lavender, sandalwood, rosemary, rose, ylang-ylang, and all citrus essential oils.

Supernatural Uses

Healer of the mind and body and spirit according to the Egyptians.[185]

- Add drops of neroli essential oil to a 1" piece of cloth or an icon of achievement when you want to achieve success in some aspect of your life. Carry it with you.

- Place a few drops of diluted neroli essential oil in your hand, rub into your palms, and inhale for courage or to face your fears.

- To bring together mind, body, and spirit use 1 drop of diluted neroli essential oil on everything, everywhere.

- Test the area or object to make sure it will not leave a stain.

- Neroli essential oil promotes congruency between heart and mind, thoughts and actions, deeds and intentions.

- Keep it around you for a few days on a cotton ball or in a pendant diffuser to help you stay aligned.

---

184 Tisserand and Young, *Essential Oil Safety*.

185 "Uses of Neroli Oil," articles.mercola.com/herbal-oils/neroli-oil.aspx.

23: Marjoram

Marjoram (*Origanum majorana*) is derived from two Greek words, *oros* (mountain) and *ganos* (joy), which is meant to capture the joyous appearance of these plants where they grow prolifically on hillsides.

Its name originates from:

Latin: *Origanum majorana*	**French:** *marjolaine*
Spanish: *mejorana*	**English:** *Marjoram, wild marjoram, sweet marjoram, garden marjoram, knotted marjoram*
Gender: *Masculine*	
Element: *Air*	
	Ruling Planet: *Mercury*

Property Description

Stimulant, carminative, diaphoretic, mildly tonic, emenagogue, analgesic, anti-spasmodic, aphrodisiac, anti-septic, anti-viral, bactericidal, cephalic, cordial, diaphoretic, digestive, diuretic, expectorant, fungicidal, hypotensive, laxative, nervine, sedative, stomachic, vasodilator, vulnerary.

Benefits

Muscle relief, headaches, circulation, respiration, infections, PMS, fungal infections, ringworm, shingles, sores.

The ancient Greeks used marjoram essential oil as a natural treatment for many ailments. They believed it helped the body heal from poison, convulsions, and edema.

Background

Marjoram boasts a very ancient medical reputation. The Greeks used it extensively, both internally and externally in poultices and compresses.[186] It was an antidote for narcotic poisons and a remedy for convulsions and dropsy. If marjoram grew on a Greek grave, it meant that the departed was happy in the afterlife. Among both the Greeks and Romans, it was the custom to crown young couples with marjoram to wish them joy and happiness.[187]

---

186   "Marjoram as an Herb" www.bellybytes.com/herbs/marjoram.html#.VpGSYY-cFaQ.

187   M. Grieve, "Marjoram, Wild," www.botanical.com/botanical/mgmh/m/marwil20.html.

Marjoram is one of the herbs associated with Samhain, a Celtic Pagan holiday that is the basis for the secular Halloween. Marjoram also has an association with spirits, as it was thought to "help the dead sleep peacefully."[188] Marjoram has been used in Sephardic Jewish tradition for healing and to divine the cause of an illness.[189]

Marjoram was believed to encourage love. Medieval women placed it around homes for its sweet fragrance and carried it around in tiny bags to attract love and to cast love spells. It was a tradition for a young woman to place marjoram under her pillow at night to reveal her future husband in her dreams.[190]

Marjoram eventually made its way to western Europe. The English used it in beer and tobacco. It adds a minty twist to snuff.

COMMON USES FOR MARJORAM ESSENTIAL OIL

- A few drops of marjoram essential oil, diluted, put on a cotton ball and held on an aching tooth frequently relieves the pain.

- **For easing measles:** drop 6 drops in a warm cup of water. Dip a cloth in the water, wring out, and apply to breakouts. (Use gloves.)

- A warm compress of marjoram essential oil is also soothing for spasms and relief from pain and heartburn.

- Diffused or inhaled over steam, a few drops of marjoram essential oil is helpful in the relief of asthma, bronchitis, coughs, headaches, tension, insomnia, sinusitis, anxiety, nervous tension, and stress. Be sure to close your eyes.

- **For a healing bath:** 5 drops of marjoram essential oil blended with 1 tsp. of carrier oil or diluted in the bath water with ¼ C Epsom salts, can be helpful with physical exhaustion, fatigue, tension, insomnia, migraines, muscular anxiety, stress, and grief.

---

188   "Oregano and Marjoram" www.readbag.com/herbsociety-factsheets-oregano-and-marjoram.

189   www.herbsociety.org.

190   "The History of Majoram," www.myspicer.com/history-of-marjoram/.

- **For a fresh bruise:** add 3–4 drops marjoram essential oil to 1 tsp. arnica cream. Rub on bruise site.

- Inhaled and diffused marjoram essential oil can lift depression.

- Dilute 1 or 2 drops marjoram essential oil and apply to the back of the neck to lessen tension and stress.

- Diffuse a few drops of marjoram essential oil before going to bed for a better night's sleep or add to a cotton ball and place near your pillow.

- Diffuse a few drops of marjoram essential oil regularly to promote healthy respiratory function.

- Massage 1 or 2 drops marjoram essential oil diluted in 1 tsp. carrier oil over the area or into the reflex points of the feet one or two times a day to provide cardiovascular support. (Use a foot reflexology chart to find the key points.)

- **Freshen sheets for a good sleep:** mix 2 C spring water with 1 tsp. baking soda. Add 15 drops of marjoram essential oil and 10 drops lavender essential oil in a spray bottle and spritz on sheets and pillow cases for a more restful sleep.

- **Relieve painful joints:** mix one drop each of lavender, marjoram, and peppermint essential oils together with 9 drops of a carrier oil and massage into affected area.

- **For meditation and a calming diffusion, mix any five of these essential oils together:** Roman chamomile, clary sage, helichrysum, lemon, melissa, marjoram, neroli, ylang-ylang, vetiver, rose, spikenard, or frankincense.

Cautions

Marjoram essential oil might cause an allergic reaction if you are allergic to basil, hyssop, lavender, mint, oregano, or sage.

Because it is a powerful oil, do not give to children under six and dilute with carrier oil for other uses in older children.

Do not use if pregnant or breastfeeding. Do not use two weeks prior to surgery.

Blends Well With
Lavender, cedarwood, Roman chamomile, lemon, orange, peppermint, rosemary, thyme, bergamot, eucalyptus, and tea tree essential oils.

Supernatural Uses
Protection against evil, wards off negativity, relieves pain of grief, promotes happiness, love, money, protection, psychic development, courage, dreams, and rituals for death.

- Anoint yourself with a few drops of diluted marjoram essential oil and legend says you will dream of your future spouse.

- Place a drop on a 1" piece of cloth and carry with you for courage. Or anoint an amulet with marjoram essential oil and carry it with you.

- Rub a drop or 2 of diluted marjoram essential oil into your palms and inhale for psychic development.

- Diffuse marjoram essential oil for relief of grief or protection or both.

- Diffuse a few drops of tea tree essential oil with marjoram essential oil to ward off colds during winter.

24: Yarrow
Yarrow essential oil *(Achillea millefolium)* is a perennial herb that is well known throughout Europe.

This herb is believed to be a remedy for a number of ailments and diseases and has other significance in European culture as well.

Its name originates from:

Latin: *Achillea millefolium*	**English:** *Milfoil, old man's pepper, soldier's woundwort, knight's milfoil, thousand weed, nose bleed, carpenter's weed, bloodwort, staunchweed, sanguinary, devil's nettle, devil's plaything, yarroway*
Spanish: *milenrama*	
French: *achillée, mille-feuille*	
Gender: *Feminine*	
Element: *Water*	**Ruling Planet:** *Venus*

Property Description

Anti-inflammatory, anti-rheumatic, anti-septic, anti-spasmodic, astringent, carminative, cicatrisant, diaphoretic, digestive, expectorant, hypotensive, stomachic, and tonic substance.

Benefits

Yarrow essential oil is beneficial in treating circulatory diseases such as varicose veins and hemorrhoids as well as certain skin diseases, wounds, burns, acne, dermatitis, colic, constipation, and infections in the digestive, urinary, and reproductive systems.

Yarrow essential oil is used to overcome colds, cramps, fevers, kidney disorders, toothaches, skin irritations, and hemorrhages, and to regulate menses, stimulate the flow of bile, and purify the blood.[191]

Yarrow essential oil is used for hair care, fevers, hypertension, indigestion, migraines, insomnia, scars, stretch marks, acne, rashes, blood pressure, and various other illnesses.

Background

Yarrow derived its Latin name from the Greek hero Achilles, the son of the sea goddess Thetis and the mortal king Peleus. Thetis, attempting to make her son immortal, dipped him into the river Styx. His mother held onto his heel, which remained untouched by the river water. That body part was his vulnerable or weak point and gave its name to the Achilles' heel as well as the anatomical Achilles tendon.

---

191   Gail Ann, "Yarrow: A Wonderful Herb for Healing and Medicine," www.spiritguidedhealer.com/herbs/yarrow.html.

Achilles was a remarkable student of the healing arts, and yarrow was his extraordinary ally. He used it to pack and treat the wounds of his comrade warriors, which is how yarrow came to be known as *militaris*.[192]

Yarrow's most famous and ancient use is in healing wounds. It was found amongst other medicinal herbs in a Neanderthal burial site in Iraq dating from around 60,000 BCE. Its claim to fame as being one of the earliest medicinal plants used by humans begins here.[193]

The Chinese used and still use the yarrow plant for divination. The I Ching (The Book of Changes) is traditionally cast with yarrow stalks that represent forces of the universe in perfect balance—yin and yang. When cast out from the thrower's hand, the yarrow sticks fall into a pattern and reveal the answers to lifelong questions. The pattern characterizes the sixty-four hexagrams of existence. Reading the pattern of the tossed sticks provides the answer to the question asked. The reader interprets the relationship of the sticks as they have fallen and thus reads the fortune.

The Anglo Saxons believed disease was a result of poisons carried on the wind. A special soup was made to ward off sickness, disease, and evil influences. The ingredients of this soup contained nine holy healing herbs, one of which was yarrow.

Before the brewing industry was regulated and mandated that hops be used as the only herb legally allowed to be brewed into beer, many different herbs were used for their flavor. Yarrow has a bitter, aromatic flavor and was the chosen herb for gruit beer, which is reputed to be more intoxicating than regular ale.[194]

Yarrow was an important herb in Native American medicine. At least forty-six American Indian tribes used yarrow for injuries and sores and found that twenty-eight ailments responded to treatments using the herb.[195]

---

192   K. Morgenstern, "History and Uses of Yarrow," www.sacredearth.com/ethnobotany /plantprofiles/yarrow.php.

193   Lucinda, "The Benefits and Uses of Yarrow," whisperingearth.co.uk/2011/09/28/the-multiple -benefits-and-uses-of-yarrow/.

194   Morgenstern, "History and Uses of Yarrow."

195   "Yarrow: The Herb of Achilles" plantyourherbs.com/yarrow-achillea-millefolium-herb -achilles.

COMMON USES FOR YARROW ESSENTIAL OIL

- **Fevers:** to break a fever or sweat it out, mix 2 drops yarrow essential oil, 1 drop ginger essential oil, and 2 drops peppermint essential oil. Diffuse or inhale blend.

- **To help with the flu:** mix 2 drops yarrow essential oil, 1 drop ginger essential oil, 1 drop tea tree essential oil, and 2 drops peppermint essential oil. Diffuse or inhale. (If you can get yourself into a bath, use this formula, mix with ¼ C Epsom salt, and bathe for 20 minutes.)

- **Tooth pain:** 1 drop diluted yarrow essential oil on a cotton ball pressed against the aching tooth should provide relief. Don't swallow. Rinse after about 10 minutes of pressured application.

- Yarrow essential oil can help strengthen blood vessels and veins. Diffuse or inhale a few drops.

- **To reduce the look of varicose veins:** mix 2 drops of yarrow essential oil and 1 drop lemon essential oil in 1 tsp. carrier oil and massage into varicose veins.

- For minor skin irritations, use a drop of diluted yarrow essential oil on a cotton ball and spot treat for acne, itching, and bug bites.

- To cool down a sunburn, blend 6 drops of yarrow essential oil with 1 tsp. carrier oil and 1 tsp. aloe vera gel. Rub on irritated skin.

- **Hair retention:** a few drops of yarrow essential oil placed in your shampoo will help stave off baldness. (Use prior to the first signs of balding.) It's also good for your hair even if you aren't balding, so add a few drops to your shampoo.

- **Edema, swelling, and inflammation:** a few drops of yarrow essential oil mixed with 1 tsp. of carrier oil in a compress applied to swollen areas can assist with inflammation pain and swelling.

- **Menstrual issues:** mix 3 drops of yarrow essential oil with 2 drops lavender essential oil, 1 drop clary sage essential oil, and 1 drop marjoram essential oil with 1 T carrier oil. Massage clockwise on abdominal area between periods (not during).[196]

Cautions

Yarrow essential oil may result in headaches and skin irritation if continually used for long periods of time in high dosages.

Avoid using during pregnancy.

Avoid using yarrow essential oil if you are on medications for blood clotting. Yarrow essential oil tends to thin the blood and may interact with blood clotting medications. Tisserand and Young recommend a dermal maximum of 8.6 percent.[197]

Blends Well With

Cedarwood, vetiver, Roman chamomile, lemongrass, myrrh, frankincense, thyme, helichrysum, lavender, and basil essential oils.

Supernatural Uses

Courage, love, psychic powers, exorcism.

- 1 drop yarrow essential oil on a 1" piece of cloth and placed under the pillow before going to bed brings a vision of the future husband or wife.

- Yarrow essential oil is used in rituals for exorcism.

- Carry a few drops of yarrow essential oil on a handkerchief or piece of cloth if you want to attract distant relations or long-lost friends. Yarrow essential oil will draw them near.

---

196 The aromatherapy massage that women performed each day *between periods* led to a significant reduction in the number of days of menstrual pain compared to the control group, and compared to the pain previously reported with no treatment. Source: Fagen PhD N.D, Zara, "Menstrual Cramps Relieved by Essential Oils," ScienceofNaturalHealth.com, http://www.scienceofnaturalhealth.com/premenstrual-menstrual-cramps-natural-remedy.html accessed 9/17/2015

197 Tisserand and Young, *Essential Oil Safety*, 243.

NINE

The Tertiary Palette of Essential Oils 25–36

Once you have started to collect essential oils and integrate them into your daily life, if you're anything like me, you will develop an even stronger curiosity about others, strange-sounding names and all. Nature is an inspiration for so many of the creative arts including painting, music, and literature. The prolific and imaginative J. K. Rowling researched unique herbal names for her Harry Potter books and gave her characters depth and intrigue. The names of certain plants fascinate me too, especially ones I had never really heard of before, like ravensara.

I also discovered that many plants I knew from my backyard had healing properties and could be used for a myriad of health and healing purposes. For example, geranium heads the tertiary palette for the healing artist's collection.

25: Geranium

The name rose geranium, *Pelargonium graveolens,* comes from the Greek *pelargos,* which means "stork." Another name for pelargonium is "stork's-bill" due to the shape of its fruit. The genus name is derived from the Greek word for crane. The word *graveolens* refers to the strong-smelling leaves. This definition is specific to *Geranium pelargonium,* also known as rose-scented geranium, the only known species of whose flower is safe for human consumption. The flowers are five-petaled and vary from pale pink to almost white; leaves may be strongly rose-scented. The leaves are the main medicinal elements in traditional medicine and are primarily used to brew a pleasant-tasting tea with a slight hint of rose.

Its name originates from:

Latin: *Pelargonium graveolens*

Spanish: *geranio de rosa*

Gender: *Feminine*

Element: *Water*

French: *géranium de rose*

English: *Rose geranium, rose-scented pelargonium, wildemalva, crane's bill*

Ruling Planet: *Venus*

Property Description

Antispasmodic, antitumoral, anti-inflammatory, anticancerous, antibacterial, antifungal, astringent, hemostatic, cicatrisant, cytophylactic, diuretic, deodorant, styptic, tonic, vermifuge, and vulnerary agent.

Benefits

Skin conditions, dermatitis, eczema, psoriasis. Improves blood flow, stimulates liver and pancreas, helps with liver detox, cleanses oily skin, infections, (ringworm) herpes, shingles, improves circulation, aids menstrual flow, balances hormones, relieves stress and depression, reduces inflammation and irritation, improves the overall health of the skin, alleviates the effects of menopause, improves circulation, boosts kidney function, and reduces blood pressure.[198]

Background

Rose geranium hails from southern Africa, but has become a cheery garden plant throughout the world. Versatile geranium essential oil not only boasts health benefits, but it is also used in making perfumes, soaps, detergents, and household products. Geranium essential oil has been described more than once as a natural perfume in its own right.

Geraniums were first brought to Europe in the seventeenth century. They are almost exclusively used for either garden color, window boxes, or for their medicinal benefits.

---

198   "Health Benefits of Geranium Esssential Oil," www.organicfacts.net/health-benefits/essential
-oils/health-benefits-of-geranium-essential-oil.html.

The rose geranium plant is vulnerable to the climate and soil in which it grows. Much like a quartz crystal that turns yellow when it grows near sulphur, the geranium takes on the characteristics of its neighbors and organic medium.

Because of that talent, geranium essential oil can range from very sweet and rosy to musty, minty, and greenish. One type of geranium oil, known as bourbon, is a distinguished perfume oil. Bourbon geranium has a rich, rosy aroma, and is cultivated and distilled exclusively on Reunion, an island in the Indian Ocean. Perfumers enjoy working with bourbon oil because of how well it assimilates with clove, sandalwood, and lavender.[199]

Geraniums originally earned their popularity in gardens and as balcony plants because of their insect repellant properties. Geranium essential oil can be found as a main ingredient in commercial insect repellant preparations, joining up with bergamot, lemon, and citronella essential oils.[200] Room sprays made with geranium essential oil help to keep your house insect free in summer.

Ancient civilizations regarded geranium essential oil as an exceptionally powerful healer, and credited it with the ability to heal fractures and even eliminate cancers.[201]

Jean Valnet, M. D., well known throughout France as a medical doctor with roots in natural medicine, used geranium essential oil to treat his patients suffering from hepatitis and fatty livers.

COMMON USES FOR GERANIUM ESSENTIAL OIL

- **For PMS relief:** blend 1 tsp. geranium essential oil in 2 oz. of carrier oil and apply to breasts to ease soreness and swelling during PMS.

- **For soft, supple skin:** add a few drops of geranium essential oil to bath water diluted in almond, coconut, or rice milk, apply to skin mixed in a carrier oil, or add a few drops to your facial cream.

---

199   "Rose Geranium Essential Oil," yellowstaressentials.wordpress.com/2011/03/12/rose -geranium-essential-oil/.

200   *Pelargonium graveolens,*" www.oilvedic.com/geranium-pelargonium-graveolens.html.

201   "Geraniums," www.oilsandplants.com/geranium.htm.

- Diffuse 3 drops of geranium essential oil to disinfect room air and create a pleasant environment.

- **Tension and stress relief:** add 3 drops of geranium essential oil to 1 tsp. of carrier oil for massage to help circulation and tonify the liver. Helps relieve tightness.

- **For cold sores:** place 1 drop of diluted geranium essential oil on a cotton swab and dab affected area.

- **As a mood balancer:** diffuse 2 to 3 drops, or place 2 drops geranium essential oil on a cotton ball or handkerchief and inhale deeply 2 to 3 times. Pause and repeat.

- **For headache and pain relief:** add 8 to 10 drops geranium essential oil mixed with 1 T Epsom salts to bath water to help relieve headache, premenstrual syndrome, stress, and tension.

- **For cellulite, PMS, and menopause:** mix 20 drops of geranium essential oil in 1 oz. of carrier oil and massage on body focusing on lower back.

- **To repel mosquitos:** diffuse 5 to 6 drops geranium essential oil mixed with 1 or 2 drops of basil and 2 drops vetiver essential oils (optional) for a strong repellent.

- **Insomnia caused by stress:** place 4 drops of geranium essential oil on a tissue or cotton ball and place inside pillow case or diffuse 2 to 3 drops of geranium essential oil.

- **For respiratory problems:** use 5 drops of geranium essential oil in a vaporizer.

- **For sore throat and tonsillitis relief:** Use 2 to 5 drops of geranium essential oil in a steam inhalation. Or, drop 2 drops of geranium essential oil in a glass of warm water and gargle. Do not swallow.

- **As an aphrodisiac:** Use 8 to 10 drops of geranium essential oil in a bath (use almond, coconut, or rice milk to disperse) or use 2 to 3 drops in a diffuser. For more variety, you can add in a few drops of patchouli essential oil or sandalwood essential oil to the diffuser.

Cautions

Geranium essential oil influences certain hormone secretions and is therefore not advised for use by pregnant women or for those who are breastfeeding.

Tisserand and Young advise a maximum dermal concentration of 17.5 percent.[202]

Blends Well With

Bergamot, basil, cedarwood, lavender, neroli, orange, lemon, ylang-ylang, clary sage, rose, sandalwood, grapefruit, and rosemary essential oils.

Supernatural Uses

Fertility, health, love protection.

It is said that snakes will not venture where geraniums grow.[203]

- Diffuse 3 to 4 drops of geranium essential oil to release negative memories, ease nervous tension, balance emotions, lift your spirit and to summon peace, well-being, and optimism.

- Use geranium essential oil to inspire natural beauty to tonify the mind and to mobilize hidden creative and emotional reserves. Inhale, diffuse, or carry drops with you on a small piece of cloth.

- Diffused, geranium essential oil helps crystalize earthly and spiritual identities.

- Use drops of geranium essential oil in spells and rituals for stirring up spirit and passion.

---

202 Tisserand and Young, *Essential Oil Safety*, 243.

203 Scott Cunningham, *Magic Herbalism: The Secret Craft of the Wise*, second edition (Saint Paul, MN: Llewellyn Publications, 1986), 144.

- Add 2 drops of geranium essential oil to a 1" piece of cloth and place under your pillow along with a photo of your beloved. This will create a love spell for the relationship.

- Make a sachet and add 3 drops of geranium essential oil for guardianship. Place sachets in areas of the house where you need protection.

- Rub a few drops of geranium essential oil above doorways and windows to ward off intruders. (Test the surface before anointing in case of staining.)

26: Melissa

Melissa essential oil (*Melissa officinalis*) is also commonly known as lemon balm and has many creative uses. The very name *melissa* is Greek for "honey bee." Melissa was originally planted next to bee hives in order to encourage the production of a more delicious honey. Melissa essential oil is considered one of the most effective medicinal-oriented essential oils in aromatherapy and exudes a unique, herbaceous, pleasing, and sweet scent.

Its name originates from:

Latin: *Melissa officinalis* **Spanish:** *Balsamo de limon/melisa/toronjil* **Gender:** *Feminine* **Element:** *Water*	**French:** *Melisse/melisse citronnelle/monarde* **English:** *Melissa (adapted from ancient sources)/lemon balm/balm/sweet balm/ sweet Mary/heart's delight/bee balm* **Ruling Planet:** *Moon*

Property Description

Antidepressant, cordial, nervine, emenagogue, sedative, antispasmodic, stomachic, antibacterial, carminative, diaphoretic, febrifuge, hypotensive, sudorific, and tonic substance.

Benefits

Melissa essential oil is used to help with symptoms of depression, colds and viruses, nervous disorders, PMS and menopause, hormonal issues, menstrual cramps, irregular periods, irritability, and depression.

It has sedative and antispasmodic properties and has been used to help alleviate anxiety, anger, aggression, and irritability in those who suffer from Alzheimer's or dementia. Helps digestive system juices and warms the respiratory system.

One study found that using a topical application of melissa essential oil diluted in a carrier helped decrease agitation in Alzheimer's patients compared to those given a placebo.[204]

Melissa essential oil was a main ingredient in the famous Carmelite Water, created by medieval Carmelite nuns to treat nervousness and headaches. Carmelite water was found to enhance the complexion because of its main ingredient, melissa essential oil.[205]

"Melissa essential oil is highly regarded as a medicinal salve, used not only for disinfection, but also for minor to moderate skin injuries. Because it shares many medicinal properties with the rest of its species, the essential oil, when mixed with one's choice of a base oil, may even be employed as a topical analgesic although its effects tend to be milder." [206]

Kurt Schnaubelt, in *Advanced Aromatherapy,* writes:

The way in which melissa essential oil combines an excellent antiviral component with a soothing but pervasive sedative power is difficult to imagine; it has to be experienced. In its complexity, power, and gentleness, melissa essential oil perfectly illustrates how nature, time after time, works better than one dimensional synthetic medicines. [207]

---

204   Clive Holmes and Clive Ballard, "Aromatherapy in Dementia," *Advances in Psychiatric Treatment*, volume 10, 2004 via apt.rcpsych.org/content/10/4/296.full, 296–300.

205   "Melissa Essential Oil Recipes," DreamingEarth.com, http://www.dreamingearth.com /blog/melissa-essential-oil-recipes/accessed 9/18/2015

206   Ibid.

207   Kurt Schnaubelt, PhD, *Advanced Aromatherapy: The Science of Essential Oil Therapy*, (Rochester, VT: Healing Arts Press, 1998),134, 188.

On a spiritual level, melissa is physically calming, uplifting, and soothing, and produces a feeling of joyfulness and revitalization. Melissa essential oil is one of my top stars for emotional and physical well-being.

Background

According to Greek mythology, Melissa was a nymph who discovered and circulated the use of honey. It is believed she gave the bees their name.[208]

A great deal of melissa essential oil sold today is actually a blend of lemongrass and citronella oils. True melissa essential oil can be identified by its own unique aroma and properties. The cost is high because it takes 3.5 to 7.5 tons of plant material to produce 1 pound of essential oil.[209] If melissa essential oil is priced too low it is likely to be adulterated in some way, and will not contain the healing properties of the true melissa essential oil.

Avicenna from ancient Persia used melissa essential oil for nervous disorders, the heart, and emotions. He also used melissa essential oil to treat anxiety, melancholy, and to strengthen and revive the vital spirit.[210] Paracelsus (1493–1541) called this herb "the Elixir of life" while John Evelyn (1620–1706) described it as "sovereign for the brain, strengthening the memory, and powerfully chasing away melancholy."[211]

Melissa (lemon balm) was initially considered a culinary spice, a windowsill herb, and a type of vegetable. Known for its limonene aroma and its mild flavor, melissa was used as an alternative to mint and lemon in peasant cuisine. It is commonly added to soups, stews, salads, and even a number of meat-based and seafood-based dishes.[212]

Melissa essential oil is very tender on the emotions. The beauty of its gentle nature is that it can bring out those same qualities in people who use it. Melissa essential oil is calming and at the same time uplifting, a source of relief for tension-induced headaches, and helps to balance the emotions.

---

208 "Melissa" www.mythindex.com/greek-mythology/M/Melissa.html.

209 Ann Clark, "Melissa Essential Oil," bewell.com.au/store/melissa-essential-oil.

210 Derek Hodges, "Melissa Essential Oil," ayurvedicoils.com/essential-oils-info-buy-purchase _melissa-essential-oil_1051.html.

211 "Melissa Essential Oil," www.essentialoils.co.za/essential-oils/melissa.htm.

212 Alexander Leon Hardt, "Lemon Balm" www.herbs-info.com/lemon-balm.

Results of a study published in an alternative medicine journal showed melissa essential oil to be effective in reducing agitation, and may have significant quality-of-life effects.[213] It is known to stimulate optimism.

COMMON USES FOR MELISSA ESSENTIAL OIL

- **Reduce stress and anxiety:** diffuse 4 drops of melissa essential oil and fill the room with calm.

- **Mood enhancer:** diffuse 4 drops of melissa essential oil and 2 drops of lemon essential oil with 1 drop bergamot essential oil to brighten your spirits.

- **Comfort for feelings of grief and vulnerability:** blend 4 drops melissa essential oil with 1 drop frankincense essential oil in 2 tsp. of a carrier oil and use as a massage oil working clockwise around the upper torso.

- **For headaches and migraines:** add 2 drops melissa essential oil to 1 tsp. jojoba or sweet almond oil and massage around forehead, temples, or neck.

- **For restful sleep:** diffuse 4 or 5 drops of melissa essential oil and inhale deeply five times. You should experience calm.

- **Ease the blues:** diffuse 3 drops melissa essential oil with 3 drops peppermint essential oil and 3 drops bergamot essential oil. You can add melissa and bergamot essential oils to 1 T of carrier oil or lotion for massage. Skip the peppermint essential oil for massage or bath.

- **For anger or resentment relief:** diffuse a blend of 2 drops of melissa essential oil, 1 drop of bergamot essential oil, and 1 drop of lavender essential oil.

- **For chronic fatigue or post-viral conditions:** diffuse 3 drops melissa essential oil, 3 drops black pepper essential oil, and 5 drops of orange essential oil.

---

213   "Melissa Essential Oil," www.anandaapothecary.com/aromatherapy-essential-oils/melissa -essential-oil.html.

- **Fatigue relief massage:** blend together 5 drops rosemary essential oil, 5 drops melissa essential oil, 5 drops neroli or basil essential oil, and 1 T carrier oil. For a bath use blend with ¼ C Epsom salts and place in bath water. Soak for 15 minutes.

- **Carpel tunnel syndrome:** blend 5 drops melissa essential oil with 5 drops lavender essential oil, 1 drop clove bud essential oil, 1 drop cinnamon bark essential oil, 1 drop black pepper essential oil. Add to a basin of warm water large enough to soak your hands and 5" above your wrists. Soak for 5 to 10 minutes.

- **Skin restoration cream:** combine ½ C shea butter and 1 T coconut oil with 1 tsp. honey and heat until combined. Cool. When cooled, blend in 20 drops melissa essential oil, 2 drops peppermint essential oil, and 5 drops each of helichrysum and sandalwood essential oils. Store in a sterilized dark glass jar and keep in a cool place. Apply twice daily.

Cautions

Pregnant women should avoid this essential oil during the initial five months of pregnancy.

It's best to use melissa essential oil in low concentrations, no more than a .9 percent dermal maximum and not use with children and infants under age two or on those with hypersensitive/diseased/damaged skin.[214]

Dilute melissa essential oil with appropriate carrier oils and/or by blending it with other essential oils before use.

Blends Well With

Basil, Roman chamomile, lavender, neroli, geranium, rose, orange, lemon, bergamot, pink grapefruit, and ylang-ylang essential oils.

Supernatural Uses

Gentleness, peace, forgiveness, love, success, healing, brings in the energy of the spirit.

---

214   Tisserand and Young, *Essential Oil Safety*, 350–351.

- Diffuse melissa essential oil for appreciation of past life lessons and for incorporating them into life today and moving forward with wisdom.

- To receive understanding and support, diffuse or inhale melissa essential oil (over steam or from rubbing into your palms) or dab a few drops on a 1" piece of cloth and put under your pillow.

- **Before meditation:** place 2 drops of melissa essential oil onto a cotton ball, sniff, and expect a spiritual awakening.

- A few drops of diluted melissa essential oil sprinkled on the body brings happiness.

27: Clove Bud

Clove bud essential oil is among the most powerful of all the aromatherapy oils. Native to the Indonesian Maluka islands, cloves were a treasured commodity prized in ancient Rome. This spice was among the first to be traded. Evidence of cloves has been found in vessels dating as far back as 1721 BCE.[215]

The Chinese also used cloves as early as 226 BCE. Those meeting the emperor would masticate flowerettes beforehand so they would not offend him with bad breath.[216]

Its name originates from:

Latin: *Syzygium aromaticum, Eugenia caryophyllata*	**Element:** *Fire*
Spanish: *Clavo de olor*	**French:** *Clou de girofle*
Gender: *Masculine*	**English:** *Clove, mykhet, carenfil*
	Ruling Planet: *Jupiter*

---

215   W. J. Rayment, "History of Cloves," www.indepthinfo.com/cloves/story.shtml.

216   Paul Muire, "Thai Beef Masaman Curry," historyofasianfood.blogspot.com/2015/08/thai -beef-massaman-curry.html.

Property Description

Analgesic, antiseptic, antispasmodic, antineuralgic, carminative, anti-infectious, disinfectant, insecticide, stimulant, stomachic, uterine, and tonic.

Benefits

Clove bud essential oil can be used for acne, bruises, burns, and cuts, keeping infection at bay and as a pain reliever. It helps with toothache, mouth sores, rheumatism, and arthritis.

It is beneficial to the digestive system, effective against vomiting, diarrhea, flatulence, spasms, and parasites, as well as bad breath.

Clove bud essential oil is valuable for relieving respiratory problems, like bronchitis, asthma, and tuberculosis.

Due to its antiseptic properties, clove bud essential oil is useful for wound, cuts, scabies, athlete's foot, fungal infections, bruises, prickly heat, scabies, and other types of injuries. It also has properties to repel moths and red fire ants. Clove bud essential oil has long been used to aid in dentistry due to its anesthetic properties.

> "Clove bud essential oil has been shown in studies to have both analgesic and antibacterial properties, which can be particularly helpful in the case of a toothache instigated by bacteria." [217]

Background

Cloves, and clove products, were one of the most precious spices of the sixteenth and seventeenth centuries. In 1522, Magellan's ship returned from its fateful trip around the world (Magellan himself died in the Philippines in 1521 at the Battle of Mactan) loaded with cloves and nutmeg, much to the delight of the Spanish.

Cloves were worth more than their weight in gold, and the Spanish crown was thrilled at the spicy treasure.

In 1605, the Dutch traders attempted to overtake and monopolize the clove trade. To corner the market, they sent ships and crews to destroy clove trees that sprouted up anywhere outside of their control.

---

217 Anaha O'Connor, "Clove Oil for Tooth Pain," well.blogs.nytimes.com/2011/02/17/remedies
-clove-oil-for-tooth-pain/comment-page-2.

The citizens of Ternate, Maluka, had been epidemic-free until the Dutch ravaged their clove trees. Unprotected, many died as a result of contagious diseases because they no longer had cloves to protect and immunize them.

Native tradition called for the planting of a clove tree to celebrate the birth of a child. The life of the tree and the child were spiritually tied together; if something happened to the tree, it did not bode well for the child. As a result of sickness and disrupted traditions, an uprising occurred and the Dutch became a loathed invader.

By the eighteenth century cloves were being grown in other places including Zanzibar, Madagascar, Brazil, Mauritius, Tidore, and Tanzania. The growth of the new supply allowed the prices to fall and cloves became affordable for all classes of people.

This spice gets its name from the French word *clou*, which means "nail," as the bud resembles a small nail when dried. The bud itself is actually the dried flower bud that grows on the branches of its evergreen tree.

Pliny praised cloves, as did the great Roman doctor Alexander Trallianus. St. Hildegarde, in her book *Morborum Causae et Gurae*, wrote that cloves were included in treatments for headaches, migraines, deafness after a cold, and dropsy (edema). She advised that cloves would warm people feeling the cold, and cool down those who felt hot. During the Renaissance, pomanders (whole oranges studded with clove buds) were made to keep epidemics and plague at bay.[218]

Common Uses for Clove Bud Essential Oil

- **Digestive problems:**
    1. Diffuse 4 or 5 drops of clove bud essential oil near the dining room before and after meals.
    2. Dilute 5 drops of clove bud essential oil with 1 T of carrier oil and massage clockwise around your abdominal area.

- **Nausea relief:** under the supervision of a certified Aromatherapist, add 1 drop of clove bud essential oil to your herbal tea to relieve the symptoms of nausea.

---

218   Daniele Ryman, "Clove Essential Oil" in *Daniele Ryman's Aromatherapy Bible*, (London: Piatkus Books, 2002.)

- **Sick room disinfectant:** diffuse 4 drops of clove bud essential oil to kill germs and purify the air.

- **Muscle aches and joint relief:** mix 8 drops of clove bud essential oil into 2 oz. of carrier oil and massage onto the affected area.

- **Toothache:** add a couple drops of diluted clove bud essential oil to a cotton swab and rub onto achy tooth for instant relief. This helps kill the infection-causing bacteria and reduces pain.

- **Throat pain:** mix 1 or 2 drops clove bud essential oil to 1 C of water. Gargle with the mixture to reduce pain. Do not swallow.

- **Bad breath help:** mix 1 or 2 drops clove bud essential oil to 1 C of water. Gargle with the mixture to clean mouth. Do not swallow.

- **Stress relief:** diffuse 4 or 5 drops clove bud essential oil or inhale over steam with your eyes closed for a stimulating effect on the mind and to remove mental exhaustion and fatigue.

- **Respiratory problems (coughs, colds, bronchitis, asthma, sinusitis):** diffuse 5 drops of clove bud essential oil to curb the inflammation.

- **Moths be gone:** place a few drops of clove bud essential oil on a cotton ball. Put the cotton ball in your closet, drawers, and linen cabinet. Not only will the fragrance spice up your closet, but it will help to send moths far away.

- **Insecticide:** combine 5 drops of clove bud essential oil with 5 drops of peppermint essential oil and 2 drops of lemon essential oil in a quart of water. Stir well. Pour the mixture into a spray bottle. Spritz the area around baseboards, under cabinets and appliances, and on countertops to repel common household pests. Reapply the mixture frequently in the summer months (once a week) and twice monthly in the winter.[219]

---

219 Katherine Barrington, "Clove Oil for Pest Control, www.ehow.com/info_12016446_clove-oil -pest-control.html.

Cautions

Do not use while pregnant or if you have a liver or kidney condition. Clove bud essential oil may interact with certain drugs. Check with your physician before using. Clove bud essential oil is very strong and should always be used in diluted form. Avoid using on children under the age of two. Do a patch test on your skin before applying this powerful essential oil as it may cause skin irritation. Tisserand and Young recommend a dermal maximum of .5 percent.[220]

Blends Well With

Bergamot, chamomile, clary sage, cedarwood, geranium, ginger, grapefruit, lavender, lemon, rose, sandalwood, and ylang-ylang essential oils.

Supernatural Uses

Protection, exorcism, love.

- 2 drops of clove bud essential oil on a 1" piece of cloth worn on your body will attract the opposite sex.

- Place 2 drops of clove bud essential oil on a sachet of lavender to comfort the bereaved and those suffering from grief or loss.

- Wear a few drops of clove bud essential oil in a diffuser necklace to protect against negative forces and purify the space around you.

- Diffuse 4 drops of clove bud essential oil to tonify the air and attract riches.

- Add 1 drop of clove bud essential oil to the largest bill in your wallet to attract money.

- Diffuse 2 drops of clove bud essential oil and 1 drop of bergamot to halt gossipers.

28: Spikenard

Spikenard *(Nardostachys jatamansi)*, also known as jatamansi, is widely used in herbal medicines. Several herbal medicinal preparations based on this plant are available in

---

220   Tisserand and Young, *Essential Oil Safety*, 255.

India and subcontinental countries.[221] There are several products on the market disguised as spikenard, namely things labeled "bhutkeshi" or "false jatamansi."[222] The real plant is native to Nepal. Spikenard is also one of the incenses used in ancient Egypt.

Its name originates from:

Latin: *Nardostachys jatamansi*	**French:** *Nard*
Spanish: *Aralia*	**English:** *Spikenard, nard, false valerian root, spiked nard, nardos pistile*
Gender: *Feminine*	
Element: *Water*	**Ruling Planet:** *Venus*

Property Description

Antibacterial, antifungal, anti-inflammatory, analgesic, antirheumatic, aromatic, carminative, depurative, diaphoretic/sudorific, skin tonic.

Benefits

The plant has a rich history of medicinal use and has been valued for centuries in Ayurvedic (Indian) and Unani (ancient Greco-Arab) systems of medicine. The rhizomes of the plant are used in the Ayurvedic system of medicine as a bitter tonic, stimulant, anti-spasmodic, and to treat hysteria, convulsions, and epilepsy. The root has been medically used to treat insomnia as well as blood, circulatory, and mental disorders. Some preparations of the plant have been used as a heptotonic, cardiotonic, analgesic, and diuretic in the Unani system of medicine. The plant is of economic importance and has been used to produce perfumes and dyes.[223]

Spikenard has been utilized since ancient times as a medicine for curing heart diseases, intellectual disabilities, urine-related problems, insomnia, etc. Famed Ayurvedic-healer, charaka, and "father of surgery" Sushruta incorporated spikenard in many me-

---

221 "Health Benefits of Spikenard Oil," www.organicfacts.net/health-benefits/essential-oils/health-benefits-of-spikenard-essential-oil.html.

222 "Spikenard," www.fragrantica.com/news/Jatamansi-or-Spikenard-2495.html.

223 "Jatamansi," www.drugs.com/npp/jatamansi.html.

dicinal essential oils, prescribed for edema, hemorrhoids, arthritis, gout, fractures, and obstinate skin diseases, mostly for external application.[224]

Spikenard essential oil is an excellent remedy for many skin ailments that are caused by bacterial infections. It has been used on wounds to protect them from bacterial infections. It is also a deodorant, a laxative, and a sedative.

Spikenard essential oil suppresses inflammation in the digestive and nervous systems, and counters irritability, nervousness, depression, stress, and emotions such as anxiety, anger, and panic. It also sedates cardiac problems. These sedating and relaxing are beneficial reliefs to insomnia.[225]

Background

The Bible contains several references to spikenard in both the Old and New Testaments. Catholics claim it represents Saint Joseph. Supportive of this connection, Pope Francis has included the spikenard in his coat of arms. The plant is also mentioned in the Song of Solomon in the Old Testament, "While the king sat at his table, my spikenard sent forth its fragrance." (1:12 Song of Solomon American Standard Version.) Spikenard essential oil was also used by ancient Roman perfumers.

> The plant is said to look like the tail of an ermine. The extracted perfume is an oil used by the Romans for anointing the head. Its great costliness is mentioned by Pliny.[226]

There are two other versions of spikenard: American spikenard, (*Aralia racemosa*) and ploughman's spikenard (*Inula conyza*), but we are not considering those here.

It is also easy to confuse spike oil with spikenard essential oil, but please be aware that spike oil comes from lavender and smells like a combination of rosemary and lavender. It is not spikenard essential oil.

---

224   Dr. Chandra Shakkar Gupta, "Jatamansi or Spikenard," www.fragrantica.com/notes /Jatamansi-or-Spikenard-108.html.

225   "Oil of Spikenard," www.unikkessential.com/spikenard-essential-oil.html.

226   James Orr, M.A., D.D., general ed., "Spikenard," www.internationalstandardbible.com.

For our purposes we are going to consider only the oil that comes from the *Nardostachys jatamansi* plant as our spikenard essential oil.

Common Uses for Spikenard Essential Oil

- Be sure to sniff test spikenard essential oil aroma to see how you respond to it emotionally and physically before diffusing.

- **Psoriasis:** blend 2 drops of spikenard essential oil with 2 drops of lavender essential oil diluted in a carrier oil and dab onto a small section of skin using a cotton ball dipped in the blend.

- **Enhance sexual energy and performance:** diffuse 4 to 5 drops of spikenard essential oil to heighten sexual connection between partners.

- **Blocked emotions:** diffuse 3 drops of spikenard essential oil and 1 drop of rose essential oil to thaw frozen emotions and open the full expression of feelings.

- **Balance menstrual cycle:** blend a couple of drops of spikenard essential oil into 1 tsp. carrier oil and massage onto abdomen using gentle clockwise strokes.

- **Relaxation:** diffuse a few drops to help settle your nerves or add to bath water along with 1 tsp. of carrier oil or 1 T Epsom salts.

- **Calming:** blend 2 drops spikenard essential oil, 4 drops rose essential oil, and 3 drops myrrh essential oil in 1 T carrier oil. Use for massage or bath. Disperse in bathwater with coconut, almond, or rice milk.

- **Laxative:** blend 3 to 4 drops of spikenard essential oil with 1 tsp. of carrier oil and massage it in a clockwise position around the abdomen. This massage technique can also be very soothing for related menstrual problems.

- **Insomnia:** diffuse 4 to 5 drops of spikenard essential oil for its calming effect on the nervous system.

- **Face and skin:** add a few drops of spikenard essential oil to your daily moisturizer or in a spray bottle with spring water and spritz on face to rejuvenate skin.

- For rough or wrinkled skin, try diluting a few drops of spikenard essential oil in some olive oil and apply as a natural moisturizer.

- **If you suffer from hemorrhoids:** blend 50 percent spikenard essential oil with 50 percent olive oil and apply on location. (Your first application may sting initially.)

- **To help reduce cholesterol:** apply 2 to 4 drops of diluted spikenard essential oil on wrists, inside elbows, or at the base of the throat two or three times daily.[227]

- **Enhance brain function:** apply 1 to 2 drops of spikenard essential oil diluted in 1 tsp. carrier oil on your forehead, temples, and mastoids (the bones just behind your ears) to help revitalize your brain.

- **Upset stomach:** apply a few drops of spikenard essential oil diluted in a carrier oil on the stomach for indigestion or nausea. Use clockwise strokes for application.

- **Body:** wear a couple drops of diluted spikenard essential oil as perfume to smell really good.

- **Wound cleaning:** to disinfect a wound and speed up healing place a drop or 2 of diluted spikenard essential oil on the wound.

Cautions

Do not use on children under six. Perform a skin test before using on yourself.

Spikenard essential oil is classified as nontoxic, nonirritating, and nonsensitizing.

It is thought to be safe to use for all skin types and is particularly good for dry or mature complexions. However, it's still best to avoid using during pregnancy.

---

227 Rebecca Park Totilo, "Spikenard Essential Oil Properties and Uses," searchwarp.com /swa453527–Uses-For-Spikenard-Essential-Oil.htm.

Blends Well With

Lavender, patchouli, vetiver, clove bud, cinnamon, ginger, clary sage, cedarwood, frankincense, geranium, lemon, and myrrh essential oils.

Supernatural Uses

Fidelity, health, luck, inner balance, courage, forgiveness.

Spikenard essential oil has a very high vibrational frequency that encourages a deep connection to one's inner spiritual self.

Its calming and settling properties bring about a deep state of meditation.

- **For good luck:** dab some spikenard essential oil on the beads of a necklace (make sure the beads can tolerate the oil) and wear for good luck and warding off disease. You can also find a container necklace and wear the oil in a pendant or charm.

- **To reveal secrets of the soul:** diffuse 3 drops of spikenard essential oil and 1 drop of myrrh essential oil. Settle back and listen to the wise voice within.

- Spikenard essential oil was used in an ancient Egyptian preparation called *kyphi*, a mixture of spikenard, juniper, myrrh, and cinnamon essential oils that was thought to appease the gods and improve meditation.[228] Also spelled *kapet*, it was one of the most popular types of temple incense in ancient Egypt and was also used as a remedy for a number of ailments.

- Place a drop of spikenard essential oil on an amulet and wear it around your neck for protection.

- Use a drop or 2 of spikenard essential oil (diluted in a carrier oil) for anointing.

- Place a drop or 2 of spikenard essential oil on two, 1" pieces of cloth. Place one under your pillow and one under your beloved's to keep each other faithful.

---

228 "Kyphi or Kapet in Ancient Eygpt," www.ancientegyptonline.co.uk/kyphi.html.

29: Benzoin

Benzoin, gum benjamin, is the sap (gum resin) of trees belonging to the Styrax species. A traditional ingredient in incense, ancient civilizations used it in fumigation and to aid respiratory problems.

It is also called friar's balsam, and the name originates from the ancient *lubān jāwī* or "frankincense from Java."[229]

Its name originates from:

Latin: *Styrax benzoin*
Spanish: *Resina benzoica*
Gender: *Masculine*
Element: *Air*
French: *Styrax benjoin*

English: *Friar's balsam, gum benjamin, gum benzoin, compound benzoin, baume benjoin, benjoin de sumatra, benjoin, benjuí, benzoe, benzoïne, loban, lohban, styrax benzoin, styrax paralleloneurum, Sumatra benzoin*
Ruling Planet: *Sun*

Property Description

Antidepressant, carminative, deodorant, disinfectant, relaxant, diuretic, expectorant, antifungal, antiseptic, antibacterial, vulnerary, astringent, anti-inflammatory, antirheumatic, sedative.

Benefits

Benzoin essential oil can be used for bronchitis, coughs, colds, wounds, acne, eczema, psoriasis, rheumatism, arthritis, scar tissue, circulation, nervous tension, stress, muscle pains, chilblains, rashes, and mouth ulcers. Benzoin essential oil's greatest benefit lies in its calming effect on the nervous and digestive systems, the warming effect on circulation problems, and the toning effect on the respiratory tract. It can also help control blood sugar which in turn can be helpful to diabetics.[230]

---

229 Albert Dietrich, "LUBĀN" in *The Encyclopaedia of Islam* 5, second ed., (Leiden, NL: Brill, 2012), 786a.

230 "Benzoin Essential Oil Information,"www.essentialoils.co.za/essential-oils/benzoin.htm.

People take benzoin by mouth for swelling (inflammation) of the throat and breathing passages. Some people apply it directly to the skin to kill germs, reduce swelling, and stop bleeding from small cuts. Benzoin is also used topically for skin ulcers, bedsores, and cracked skin. In dentistry, benzoin is used for swollen gums and herpes sores in the mouth. In manufacturing, benzoin is used in making pharmaceutical drugs. [231]

Background

The benjamin gum tree is native to Java, Sumatra, and Thailand and grows to 20 feet. When the tree is at least seven years old, deep incisions are made in the trunk, and the sap is extracted. When the resinous lump becomes hard and brittle, it is collected from the bark.

There are two common kinds of benzoin resin: benzoin Siam and benzoin Sumatra. Benzoin Siam is obtained from *Styrax tonkinensis*, found across Thailand, Laos, Cambodia, and Vietnam. Benzoin Sumatra is obtained from *Styrax benzoin*, which grows predominantly on the island of Sumatra.[232] Benzoin Siam(*Styrax tonkinensis*), is used only in manufacturing and *not* as a healing treatment.

Benzoin essential oil has been in use for thousands of years. Traces of its use date back to Egyptian civilization in the tomb of Hatshepsut. It has been used for centuries in Arab countries for religious and ritual uses.[233] Arabian traders brought benzoin to Greece, Rome, and Egypt where it became prized as a fixative in perfumes and potpourris—still one of its uses today. The Crusaders carried benzoin into Europe to scent their cherished Oriental type perfume. Europeans highly regarded benzoin for its medicinal properties as well as its scent.[234]

---

231   "Benzoin," www.webmd.com/vitamins-supplements/ingredientmono-351-BENZOIN.aspx ?activeIngredientId=351&activeIngredientName=BENZOIN.

232   Karl-Georg Fahlbusch et al. "Flavors and Fragrances," Ullmann's Encyclopedia of Industrial Chemistry, 7th ed., (Weinheim, Ger: Wiley-VCH, 2007), 87.

233   Balasubramanian Narayanaganesh, Center for Protease Research, Department of Chemistry and Biochemistry, North Dakota State University, NDSU Chemical Technology in Antiquity, 219–244, 2015, ACS Symposium Series, Vol. 1211, DOI: 10.1021/bk-2015–1211, ch008.

234   Kathy Keville, "Aromatherapy: Benzoin," health.howstuffworks.com/wellness/natural -medicine/aromatherapy/aromatherapy-benzoin.htm.

Most of the world's benzoin resin is used in the Arab States and India, where it is placed on hot charcoal and burned as incense. Benzoin resin is also used in blended types of Japanese, Indian, and Chinese incense.

Benzoin resin is a common ingredient in incense making and perfumery because of its sweet vanilla-like aroma and fixative properties. Gum benzoin is a major component of the incense used in churches in Russian/Eastern Orthodox as well as western Catholic churches, where it's known as St. Alban's blend.[235]

In Malaysia, benzoin essential oil is used to deter bad spirits. In Java, fishermen use benzoin essential oil before entering the dark coastal caves where fish gather.[236]

Common Uses for Benzoin Essential Oil

- **Red or itchy skin:** blend 3 drops of benzoin essential oil with 1 tsp. of carrier oil and massage into skin.

- **To extend the life of other essential oils:** benzoin essential oil acts as a strong preservative. Add it to other oils and oil-based preparations to delay oxidation and increase shelf life.

- **Lung and sinus healing:** add 12 drops of benzoin essential oil to 1 oz. of a chest rub balm and work into sinus and chest areas.

- **General aches and pains:** add 3 drops of benzoin essential oil to bath water dispersed in almond, coconut, or rice milk or 4 drops mixed in 1 oz. carrier oil for a relieving massage

- **Chronic bronchitis:** diffuse 3 to 4 drops of benzoin essential oil in a small room to ease chronic bronchitis and coughing.

- **For poor circulation:** use 3 to 4 drops benzoin essential oil in a 2 oz. carrier oil blend. Massage in a direction toward the heart.

- **Stiff muscles:** use the above blend to increase circulation by massaging into stiff and painful muscles.

---

235   St. Alban blend.

236   Valerie Ann Worwood, *Aromatherapy for the Soul: Healing the Spirit with Fragrances and Essential Oils* (San Francisco: New World Library, 2012), 205.

- **Depression:** diffuse 4 to 5 drops of benzoin essential oil to ease feelings of despondency.

- **Skin care:** mix 4 drops of benzoin essential oil into your night cream for a skin boost to increase elasticity, and reduce redness, irritation, and itchiness.

- Blend 5 drops of benzoin essential oil and 2 drops lavender essential oil with 2 oz. sweet almond oil for dry, cracked skin and cuts and wounds.

Cautions

Do not use on children under two years.

Do not use large amounts of benzoin essential oil. Do not exceed a dermal maximum of 2 percent.[237] Do not operate heavy machinery if you have used large amounts of benzoin essential oil.

Blends Well With

Sandalwood, rose, bergamot, frankincense, myrrh, palo santo, lemon, melissa, lavender, lemon, and sandalwood essential oils.

Supernatural Uses

Provides focus, guidance, protection, purification, comfort, and attracts business.

Spiritually, benzoin holds the energies and fire of sunlight. It is a joyous gift from the plant world. It comforts and cushions the soul allowing it to receive from the spirit.[238]

- Benzoin essential oil is used in rituals for Imbolc and the Autumnal Equinox.

- **For business prosperity:** use a blend of 4 drops basil essential oil, 7 drops benzoin essential oil, and 4 drops cinnamon essential oil in a diffuser, or in a bath dispersed in coconut, almond, or rice milk, or as a perfume or sachet diluted in a carrier oil.

---

237 Tisserand and Young, *Essential Oil Safety*, 210.

238 Debra Mauldin, C. A., "Healing Magical and Spiritual Properties of Essential Oils, Fragrances, Oils and Herbs II, mauldinfamily1.wordpress.com/aromatherapy-information-about/spiritual -and-magical-properties-of-essential-oils/.

- **For protection:** add 2 drops of benzoin essential oil to a cotton ball and apply to doors and windows. (Be sure to do a test before use to make sure it will not stain.)

- **To open the spirit:** diffuse 3 to 4 drops of benzoin essential oil and breathe in for 10–12 minutes. Allow the scent to open your mind and heart to the unseen gifts of the cosmos.

- To connect to forces beyond the world as we know it, diffuse 4 to 5 drops of benzoin essential oil and sit in silence allowing yourself to connect to cosmic energies.

30: Ravensara

There are two oils on the market that have similar names and claims. For our purposes we are going to consider only ravensara, not ravintsara.

Its name originates from:

Latin: *Ravensara aromatica*	**French:** *Ravensara aromatica*
Spanish: *Ravensara aromatica*	**English:** *Ravensara*
Gender: *Feminine*	**Ruling Planet:** *Moon/ Mercury*
Element: *Water/Air*	

Property Description

Analgesic, antibacterial, antimicrobial, antidepressant, antifungal, antiseptic, antispasmodic, antiviral, aphrodisiac, disinfectant, diuretic, expectorant, relaxant, tonic.

Benefits

Ravensara essential oil is relaxing and analgesic, and can be used in massage blends or compresses to relieve muscle aches and pains, strains and sprains. It will help to boost your immunity during stressful times when the body's defenses are down.

It is used for herpes zoster virus control, pain management, cold sore relief, congestion relief, prevention from colds and flu, chronic fatigue syndrome relief, mental uplift, and muscle strain release.[239]

Background

Ravensara essential oil is a powerful oil from Madagascar, the mysterious island off the eastern coast of Africa. The ravensara (botanical name *Ravensara aromatica*) is a large indigenous rainforest tree. In Madagascar, this genus of trees is commonly called *Hazomanitra,* meaning "tree that smells." The essential oil is extracted from the ravensara's leaves and is used for its medicinal properties. It is praised in Madagascar as a "cure all" oil in much the same way as tea tree oil is lauded in Australia.[240]

Ravensara essential oil holds an elevated place in Madagascar's indigenous medicinal treatment system. This oil has been used as a tonic and for fighting infections for centuries, and modern studies have revealed many other associated medicinal benefits.

Ravensara essential oil is an exceptionally powerful antiviral essential oil. It is effective when blended with *Calophyllum inophyllum* (large evergreen tree),[241] in the reduction of pain associated with the inflammation of shingles. Blended with *calophyllum*, it has been successfully used to treat all forms of herpes.

Common Uses for Ravensara Essential Oil

- **For herpes or shingles:** ravensara essential oil is an anti-viral and has been quite effective in getting rid of herpes and shingles lesions.[242] Mix 4 drops of ravensara essential oil with 3 drops of tea tree essential oil. Add 1 T of

---

239 "Ravensara Oil for Cold Sores, Shingles and Herpes," www.essentialoilexchange.com/blog /ravensara-oil-for-cold-sores-shingles-and-herpes/.

240 "Health Benefits of Ravensara Essential Oil," www.organicfacts.net/health-benefits/essential -oils/health-benefits-of-ravensara-essential-oil.html.

241 *Calophyllum inophyllum* is a large evergreen, commonly called Alexandrian laurel balltree, beach calophyllum, beach touriga, beautyleaf, Borneo-mahogany, Indian doomba oiltree, Indian-laurel, laurelwood, satin touriga, and tacamahac-tree. It is native to East Africa and the southern coast of India.

242 "Ravensara Essential Oil," oilhealthbenefits.com/ravensara-essential-oil/.

carrier oil like aloe vera gel, tamanu, or coconut oil. Apply this blend using a cotton ball on cold sores, genital herpes, and shingles lesions. Reapply two times a day for relief from the pain and soreness.

- **Clear up phlegm and mucous:** inhale the vapors of ravensara essential oil by putting a few drops of it in boiling water, covering your head with a towel, and closing your eyes to inhale the vapors.

- **Colds, flu, and congestion:** at the first sign of a cold, use a bath treatment and/or steam inhalation treatment and rub 2 drops of ravensara essential oil on feet blended with 2 drops of tea tree essential oil in a carrier base of 1 tsp. For the bath disperse in Epsom salts, almond, rice of coconut milk.

- **For despair:** inhale or diffuse the aroma of ravensara essential oil. This treatment will subdue melancholy and will uplift the heart and mind.

- **For a broken heart:** diffuse 3 drops of ravensara essential oil, 2 drops of rose, 1 drop of frankincense, 1 drop of melissa, 1 drop of helichrysum, 1 drop eucalyptus, and 2 drops of bergamot essential oils.

- **To boost the immune system:** blend 3 drops each of ravensara essential oil with rosemary, tea tree, and eucalyptus essential oils in 2 T carrier oil. Inhale or use for massage.

- **For bacterial infections:** ravensara essential oil is a powerful antibacterial agent. It can kill *H. pylori,* a strain that afflicts the stomach and leads to a host of digestive problems.[243] For internal treatment see a certified Aromatherapist.

- **To soothe sore muscles:** add 10 to 15 drops of ravensara essential oil to your bath dispersed in almond, coconut, or rice milk and soak for about 15 minutes to bring relief to sore, painful, and aching muscles.

---

243 "Ravensara Essential Oil," oilhealthbenefits.com/ravensara-essential-oil/.

A warm water bath with ravensara essential oil also alleviates nervous tension and promotes sleep.

- **Chronic fatigue syndrome relief:** place 2 drops of ravensara essential oil on a cotton ball and place under nose. Inhale for 5 to 10 minutes. This should increase energy and relieve chronic pain. Do not do this procedure more than six times a day.

- **Headaches:** diffuse 4 to 5 drops of ravensara essential oil to purify the air and distribute its mild scent.

- **For sinus and nasal congestion:** either diffuse as above, or place 4 drops of ravensara essential oil into a pot of steaming water, place a towel over your head, close your eyes, and inhale vapors for 5 to 10 minutes. This will help to reduce congestion in the sinuses and the nose.

- **Reduce stress:** diffuse or inhale 4 to 5 drops of ravensara essential oil. The aroma relaxes the body.

- **Stress relief massage:** blend 3 drops of ravensara essential oil with 2 drops of chamomile essential oil and 2 drops of lavender essential oil in 2 oz. of a carrier oil to lower physical stress on the muscles.

- **For mental stress relief:** blend 3 drops of ravensara essential oil with 2 drops of chamomile essential oil and 2 drops of spikenard essential oil in 2 oz. of a carrier oil to provide relief. Use for massage.

Cautions

There are no contraindications for ravensara except the normal precautions for using essential oils. Tisserand and Young recommend only using oil from the leaf and not the bark oil. Keep to a dermal maximum of .12 percent. They also advise to use this product under the supervision of a qualified Aromatherapist.[244]

---

244   Tisserand and Young, *Essential Oil Safety*, 403.

Blends Well With

Bergamot, black pepper, clary sage, cedarwood, eucalyptus, frankincense, geranium, ginger, grapefruit, lavender, lemon, marjoram, rosemary, sandalwood, tea tree, and thyme essential oils.

Supernatural Uses

Cleansing, healing, mind-clearing, stimulates courage.

- **To relieve grief:** place 3 drops of ravensara essential oil on a cotton ball, wrap in a linen handkerchief, and breath in as you repeat "I allow myself this moment and I move through it with love and acceptance. All is well." Carry the cotton ball with you to remind you of this affirmation. Repeat: "Love and time will heal me."

- **To contact angels:** diffuse 3 drops of ravensara, 3 drops of neroli, and 2 drops of frankincense essential oils. Allow the aromas to permeate the room and sit in silence and meditation. Angels will come.

- **To forgive:** blend 2 drops of ravensara essential oil with 1 drop each of frankincense, melissa, and spikenard essential oil. Mix with 1 T of carrier oil and use this as an application for your heart and your feet. Sit in silence and picture yourself as whole and healed. The mantra is: "Forgive, but don't forget." Find the way to balance those thoughts within yourself.

- **Learn to love again:** diffuse 4 drops of ravensara essential oil and meditate for 15 minutes on your healthy heart, your greatest joys, and something that brings peace into your soul. Focus on those things as you intake the aromas.

31: Cedarwood

Like many oils derived from the pine or cypress botanical family, cedarwood essential oil is anti-bacterial and pesticidal. It has many uses in medicine, art, industry, and perfumery. The essential oil is processed from the foliage, wood, and roots of conifers.

Cedarwood essential oil was used in Egypt as an ingredient in a poison antidote called *mithridat,* and may well have been the first essential oil to ever be extracted. It was used throughout the East for bronchitis and other respiratory infections.[245]

Its name originates from:

Latin: *Juniperus Virginia, Cedrus Doedara, Cedrus Atlantica,* or *Cedrus Libani,* depending on the regions where they are found. **Spanish:** *Madera de cedro* **Gender:** *Masculine*	**Element:** *Fire* **French:** *bois de cèdre* **English:** *Cedarwood* **Ruling Planet:** *Sun*

Property Description

Antiseborrheic, antiseptic, antispasmodic, tonic, astringent, diuretic, emenagogue, expectorant, insecticide, sedative, fungicide.

Benefits

Cedarwood essential oil calms nervous tension and anxiety, promotes sleep, relaxes tight muscles, helps ease muscle and joint pain, supports breathing when used as an inhalation, and is helpful in meditation.

It is mildly astringent, good for acne, oily skin and hair, dandruff, hair loss, and may help reduce cellulite. It is fungicidal and a powerful insect repellant.

Due to its positive effects on the scalp, cedarwood essential oil may also have a helpful effect on alopecia and premature balding.

In a recent study, subjects applied a blend of thyme, rosemary, cedarwood, and lavender essential oils in a base of jojoba or grapeseed oil to the scalp. The group using essential oils showed significant improvement.[246]

---

245   Julia Lawless, *The Encyclopedia of Essential Oils: The Complete Guide to the Use of Aromatic Oils In Aromatherapy, Herbalism, Health, and Well Being* (San Francisco: Conari Press, 2013).

246   "Cedar Oil," www.anandaapothecary.com/aromatherapy-essential-oils/cedar-atlas-essential -oil.html.

Cedarwood essential oil may help with the symptoms of ADHD. A study performed by Dr. Terry Friedmann and Dennis Eggett from Brigham Young University found that using cedarwood essential oil on children could greatly improve their focus and learning capacity.

Thirty-four children with ADHD were given different single essential oils including vetiver, cedarwood, lavender, and an oil blend. Children held up a bottle of essential oils and took three deep inhalations three times a day for thirty days. At the end of the study, subjects retook an EEG and T.O.V.A. test—with both vetiver and cedarwood essential oils there were significant changes. The results showed cedarwood essential oil inhalation improved focus in children with ADHD by 65 percent.[247]

Background

The original sources of ancient cedarwood essential oil were the precious cedars of Lebanon, native to the mountains in the Middle East. Due to rampant overharvesting, those cedars are long gone, and none of the oil in use today is produced from the original Lebanese cedars.

The ancient Sumerians used cedarwood essential oil as a base for paints, and in India, oil from the deodar cedar (*Cedrus deodorata*) has been used for its insecticidal and anti-fungal properties.

It appears that while the Sumerians were painting with it and the Indians were running off insects with cedarwood essential oil, the Egyptians were using it for embalming. It tendered double duty: an effective preservative that also kept insects from disturbing the mummified body.

One out of three methods of ancient Egyptian embalming practices employed the use of cedarwood essential oil. This alternative was a less costly method than the most familiar of ancient Egyptian practices of removing internal organs and placing them in separate canopic jars for preservation.[248]

---

247   Josh Axe, MD, draxe.com/cedarwood-essential-oil/.

248   "Egyptian Afterlife." www.crystalinks.com/egyptafterlife.html.

Even today, cedarwood essential oil is still in high demand. The oil products come from the Atlas Mountains, (*Cedrus atlantica*), North America, (*Cedrus virginiana*, closely related to *Juniperus virginiana*), and India (*Cedros deodara*).[249] The trees grow in cold climates and high altitudes.

COMMON USES FOR CEDARWOOD ESSENTIAL OIL

- **For eczema:** add 2 to 3 drops of cedarwood essential oil to your skin lotion or liquid body soap. Rub it on the infected or itchy area directly. You can also make a skin-helping bath using five drops of cedarwood essential oil added to the bath water. Soak for at least 10 to 15 minutes.

- **Hair loss prevention:** add 5 drops of cedarwood essential oil to your shampoo or conditioner, or just massage the oil into your scalp and let it sit for 30 minutes before rinsing.

- **Dry scalp:** mix 2 drops of cedarwood essential oil with 1 T fractionated coconut oil for antifungal and moisturizing properties. Rub mixture into your scalp for 5 minutes. Let sit for 20 to 30 minutes and then rinse out.

- **Relief for restless leg and muscle spasms:** diffuse 4 to 5 drops of cedarwood essential oil to ease the cramping and tightness. Dilute 5 drops of cedarwood essential oil in 1 tsp. of carrier oil and massage sore or tight muscles. Massage your abs, arms, chest, and legs. You should experience a soothing and fresh sensation.

- **Mosquito and insect repellant:** place a few drops of diluted (3 drops to 1 tsp.) cedarwood essential oil on your skin to keep mosquitos away outdoors. A diffuser will help keep them out of the house. Also try a

---

249 *Juniperus virginiana*—common names include red cedar, eastern red-cedar, eastern redcedar, eastern juniper, red juniper, pencil cedar, and aromatic cedar—is a species of juniper native to eastern North America from southeastern Canada to the Gulf of Mexico and east of the Great Plains. Further west it is replaced by the related *Juniperus scopulorum* (Rocky Mountain Juniper) and to the southwest by *Juniperus ashei* (Ashe Juniper). Ref: Farjon, A. (2005). Monograph of Cupressaceae and Sciadopitys. Royal Botanic Gardens, Kew.

mix of water (1 C) and 6 drops of cedarwood essential oil to spray on your bed and furniture to repel the bugs.

- **Moth repellant:** apply a few drops of cedarwood essential oil to cotton balls and place them in your closet, on your hangers and inside of storage boxes.

- **Reduce stress and relieve depression:** inhale cedarwood essential oil directly from the bottle; you can also diffuse a few drops of oil or rub a drop of diluted cedarwood essential oil 1 inch above your eyebrows to relieve tension.

- **Mild acne relief:** add 1 drop of cedarwood essential oil to your lotion or face soap. Use daily.

- **Exfoliating face scrub:** mix 2 drops cedarwood essential oil, 1 T Epsom salt, and 1 T fractionated coconut oil together until you get a rough texture. Use as a face scrub for your skin and to clear up acne.

- **Blonde hair special rinse:** mix 15 drops cedarwood essential oil and 10 drops lemon essential oil into 8 oz. hair conditioner. This blend keeps hair shiny-bright.

Cautions
Best avoided during pregnancy.

Blends Well With
Bergamot, Roman chamomile, clary sage, eucalyptus, frankincense, geranium, pink grapefruit, lavender, marjoram, neroli, orange, rosemary, sandalwood, vetiver, and ylang-ylang essential oils.

Supernatural Uses
Healing, purification, money, protection.

- **To alleviate bad dreams:** diffuse 4 to 5 drops of cedarwood essential oil before going to sleep. (Add 1 drop of rose for happy dreams.)

- **For physical protection:** dab a few drops of cedarwood essential oil above the doorway and on windowsills to ward off lightning and bad weather. (Pre-check for staining.)

- Need more cash? Place 1 drop cedarwood essential oil onto a 1" square cloth and carry in your wallet to attract money.

- Add a few drops of cedarwood essential oil to a sachet to induce psychic powers.

32: Cinnamon

Four thousand years ago, cinnamon was used in perfumes.[250] The ancient Chinese used cinnamon essential oil for food preparation and medicinal purposes dating as far back as 2800 BCE.

Cinnamon's name is derived from the Phonecians. The Greeks called it *kinnámmon*, but the botanical name for the spice *Cinnamomum zeylanicum* is derived from Sri Lanka's former (colonial) name, Ceylon.

Cinnamon trees grow in India and Sri Lanka. Cinnamon essential oil is yielded from the bark and leaves of the cinnamon tree. The oil harvested from the leaves is less expensive, whereas the oil gleaned from the bark is more potent and effective.

Its name originates from:

Latin: *Cinnamomum verum, Cinnamomum zeylanicum*	**French:** *Canelle*
Spanish: *Canela*	**English:** *cinnamon, sweet wood, Ceylon cinnamon*
Gender: *Masculine*	**Ruling Planet:** *Sun*
Element: *Fire*	

---

250   "Cinnamon Essential Oil," www.cinnamon-oil.net/cinnamon-oil-uses.html.

Property Description

Analgesic, antiseptic, antibiotic, antispasmodic, aphrodisiac, astringent, cardiac, carminative, emenagogue, insecticide, stimulant, stomachic, tonic, vermifuge.

Benefits

Cinnamon essential oil is useful for relieving sore throats, coughs, sneezing, and mild headaches.

Cinnamon essential oil has also been used for flatulence, nausea, diarrhea, and painful menstrual periods. It's also believed to improve energy, vitality, and circulation, and to be particularly useful for people who tend to feel hot in their upper body but have cold feet.

In Ayurveda, cinnamon essential oil is used as a remedy for diabetes, indigestion, and colds, and it is often recommended for people with the kapha dosha Ayurveda type.[251]

Due to its very powerful antiseptic properties it is good for fighting any infectious disease. It also has great value for calming spasms of the digestive tract, nausea, and vomiting. It stimulates secretion of digestive juices, while easing muscular and joint pains associated with rheumatism and arthritis. Care should be taken not to irritate the skin and mucous membranes.[252]

Recent scientific research has revealed that cinnamon essential oil offers many health benefits and can be used to treat many ailments that plague the common man. Cinnamon essential oil has powerful antibacterial and anti-cancer properties. A research study published in *Food and Chemical Toxology* in November 2010 identified nine active agents in cinnamon essential oil. The essential oil effectively hindered the activities of twenty-one species of bacteria and four *Candida* fungus species. This research study demonstrated the capability of cinnamon essential oil in the prevention and cure of some infections and some types of cancer.[253]

Research studies also showed the ability of cinnamon essential oil to prevent or reduce inflammation. The study showed the anti-inflammatory effects of cinnamon essential oil extracted from the leaves of the plant where the extract inhibited nitric oxide, the chemical

---

251 "Cinnamon," spavelous.com/EB/N071207/Holiday2.html.

252 "Cinnamon Leaf Oils," www.essentialoils.co.za/essential-oils/cinnamon-leaf.htm.

253 "Cinnamon Oil Uses," www.cinnamon-oil.net/cinnamon-oil-uses.

substance that triggers inflammation. The cinnamon essential oil also inhibited lipid oxidation and the immune system activity associated with atherogenic plaque formation. The study concluded that cinnamon essential oil has significant anti-inflammatory properties and can be used as a natural anti-inflammatory agent.[254]

Published in the April 2010 issue of *Molecules*, a medical journal, cinnamon essential oil was shown to be the best anti-bacterial substance that can inhibit *P. acnes,* the bacteria that causes acne. "At 5 percent concentration of cinnamon oil, all the P. acnes bacterial were killed in a span of 5 minutes." In addition, this study also showed that cinnamon oil has more toxicity to human prostate cancer cells than breast or lung cancer cells.[255]

One teaspoon of cinnamon powder has as much antioxidant capacity as a full cup of pomegranate juice or a half-cup of blueberries.[256]

Background

There are two kinds of cinnamon essential oil on the market. One is made from the bark and one is made from the leaves of the tree. The bark product has a sweet, pungent, and delicate aroma. The leaf product has a stronger odor when compared to the bark oil.[257] (See more notes under Cautions.) You can use the leaf or the bark variety. I prefer the bark oil for healing and the leaf for diffusing and scenting the house.

Avoid cassia cinnamon essential oil. It is the less expensive variety and the type of common cinnamon (powder) sold in supermarkets. This variety grows on small trees in India, Sri Lanka, Indonesia, Brazil, Vietnam, and Egypt. It has a darker color.

In the Old Testament and Hebrew Bible, there is a notation that Moses prescribed cinnamon essential oil for anointing. In Proverbs (7:17) it is described as a perfume. It is also

---

254   "Cinnamon Oil Uses," www.cinnamon-oil.net/cinnamon-oil-uses.

255   Ibid.

256   "Cinnamon Oil Benefits Come from Come from Its High Antioxidant Content," www
      .antioxidants-for-health-and-longevity.com/cinnamon-health-benefits.html.

257   Cinnamon bark oil is a more expensive variety when compared to cinnamon leaf oil. The
      entire tree has to be harvested to get the bark whereas leaves are more easily plucked without
      damaging the tree. "Difference Between Cinnamon Bark Oil and Cinnamon Leaf Oil," www
      .benefitsfromcinnamon.com/general-info/difference-between-cinnamon-bark-oil
      -and-cinnamon-leaf-oil.

mentioned in the Psalms (48:8), Exodus (30:23), John (19:39), and in Song of Solomon (4:14) describing the beauty of his beloved, "cinnamon scents her garments like the smell of Lebanon." [258]

Once called "the emperor of spices," cinnamon and cinnamon essential oil was so highly prized that it was fit to be gifted to kings and gods alike. In ancient Egypt cinnamon and cinnamon essential oil was used medicinally and as a flavoring for beverages. It was generously used in embalming, where body cavities were filled with spicy preservatives. Due to the variety of its uses in the ancient world, cinnamon essential oil was more precious than gold. [259]

Cinnamon essential oil was popular in ancient anointing rituals. Wreaths of cinnamon leaves decorated Roman temples. Cinnamon has a refreshing aroma and to this day is extensively used in making perfumes.

In the middle ages, cinnamon (spice and essential oil) was only affordable by the wealthy elite. In fact, it was easy to deduce a person's social rank during that time by counting the number of spices that person could afford.

From the sixteenth to the nineteenth centuries, there were power struggles among European nations over who would control Ceylon and the lucrative cinnamon industry. So much so that the rise of the West in modern times can be partly attributed to cinnamon. The West colonized Asia in part to grow spice trees and plants, harvest them, and ship them to Europe.

Consumer demand for cinnamon was a large enough market to launch several merchant enterprises for the explorers of the day. The Portuguese invaded Sri Lanka immediately after reaching India in 1536, and forced the Sinhalese king to pay the Portuguese tributes (ransom) of 110,000 kilograms of cinnamon annually. [260]

---

258   "Cinnamon," www.cryofoods.com/spice-for-life-encyclopedia.asp.

259   "Cinnamon," www.agriculturalproductsindia.com/spices/spices-cinnamon.html.

260   Ibid.

Common Uses for Cinnamon Essential Oil

- **For arthritis and joint relief:** mix one part honey to two parts lukewarm water with 1 tsp. of cinnamon powder. Add 3 drops of cinnamon essential oil. Make a paste and massage it on the swollen and painful joint or part of the body. The pain should begin to recede within a minute or two.

- To alleviate a bladder infection, mix 1 drop of cinnamon essential oil into a glass of lukewarm water mixed with 1 tsp. honey. This warm drink helps destroy germs in the bladder. Because cinnamon essential oil is powerful and an irritant be sure to only do this under the supervision of a certified Aromatherapist.

- **Acne and skin problems:** mix 3 drops of cinnamon essential oil with 3 T of honey and 1 tsp. of cinnamon powder. Apply this paste onto pimples, allow to set for 20 minutes, then wash with warm water.

- **For a room freshener:** add a few drops of cinnamon essential oil to a mist bottle filled with 1 C distilled water and spray the room.

- **Instant warmer:** diffuse 3 drops of blended cinnamon bark, 2 drops sandalwood, and 2 drops clove bud essential oils.

- **Autumn inspired room mist:** combine 4 oz. water, 4 oz. witch hazel, 20 drops cinnamon, 15 drops ginger, 15 drops clove bud, 15 drops orange, 6 drops sandalwood, and 5 drops bergamot essential oils into a 16 oz. glass spray bottle. Shake well and mist room for a warm and cozy harvest atmosphere.

- **As a remedial room spray:** mix 8 drops of cinnamon essential oil with 7 oz. water and 1 oz. vodka in a spray mist bottle. Spritz the room when you want to dispel strong odors.

- **For respiratory problems:** diffuse a small amount, 1 to 2 drops of cinnamon essential oil, in the room as a reliever of colds, flu, influenza, and other respiratory problems.

Cautions

Cinnamon leaf essential oil, which is extracted from the leaf, is nontoxic. However large amounts inhaled may cause damage to mucous membranes. Both varieties are dermal irritants, mucous membrane irritants, and sensitizers. Of the two cinnamon essential oil varieties available, highly diluted cinnamon leaf is the essential oil most commonly used in aromatherapy. Follow safety precautions and dilution guidelines before using. Speak with your doctor before using any of these cinnamon essential oils if you are taking medications for blood thinning or diabetes.

Cinnamon bark essential oil is very strong and should not be used directly on the skin. It has powerful anti-fungal and anti-bacterial properties and can be used as a diffuser in aroma lamps to cleanse the air. It can also cause sensitization and irritation if used in too strong a dose. Robert Tisserand recommends a 1 percent dilution for cinnamon essential oils. That translates into 1 drop in 30/40 ml of a carrier oil.[261]

Blends Well With

Benzoin, clove bud, frankincense, myrrh, lemongrass, vetiver, ginger, pink grapefruit, lavender, rosemary, and thyme essential oils.

Supernatural Uses

Spirituality, success, healing, power, psychic powers, lust, protection, love.

- A few drops of cinnamon essential oil diffused can raise spiritual vibration. Use before meditation or doing or receiving a psychic reading.

- Add a few drops of cinnamon essential oil to sachets and carry as protection.

- Put a few drops of cinnamon essential oil on a 1" piece of cloth and carry in your wallet to attract money to you.

- Use diluted (1 drop cinnamon essential oil to 10 drops of jojoba or almond oil) for anointing, consecrating, and initiating.

---

261   Robert Tisserand, "New Survey Reveals Dangers of Not Diluting Essential Oils," tisserandinstitute.org/new-survey-reveals-dangers-of-not-diluting-essential-oils/.

33: Lemongrass

Most of the species of lemongrass are native to south and southeast Asia and Australia. The so-called east Indian lemongrass (*Cymbopogon flexuosus*), also known as Malabar or Cochin grass, is native to India, Sri Lanka, Burma, and Thailand. Both members of the species are cultivated today throughout tropical Asia.

Lemongrass is widely used as a culinary herb in Asia and is common as a dried powder in soups, curries, and teas for its subtle citrusy flavor. In India it is mostly used as a medicinal herb.[262]

Its name originates from:

Latin: *Cymbopogon citratus*	**French:** *Citronnelle*
Spanish: *Hierba de limón*	**English:** *Lemongrass, barbed wire grass, silky heads, citronella grass, fever grass*
Gender: *Masculine*	
Element: *Air*	
	Ruling Planet: *Mercury*

Property Description

Analgesic, antidepressant, antimicrobial, antipyretic, antiseptic, astringent, bactericidal, carminative, deodorant, diuretic, febrifuge, fungicidal, insecticidal, nervine, sedative, tonic.

Benefits

Lemongrass essential oil helps relieve body pain related to strenuous activities. It can also alleviate symptoms of toothaches, headaches, and viral infections from cough, cold, influenza, and fever.[263]

Lemongrass essential oil has been found to boost self-esteem, confidence, hope, and mental strength. It also can relieve anxiety.

---

262   Namita Nayyar, "Lemongrass: A Multi-beneficial Herb," www.womenfitness.net/lemongrass_beneficialHerb.htm.

263   "Health Benefits of Lemongrass Oil," www.organicfacts.net/health-benefits/essential-oils/health-benefits-of-lemongrass-essential-oil.html.

It has many therapeutic properties and is used extensively in Ayurvedic medicine. It is helpful in relieving cough and nasal congestion.[264]

Background

Lemongrass essential oil was found to be used as a pesticide and a preservative. Early manuscripts in India were found to have been treated with lemongrass essential oil as a prophylactic measure against humidity, decay, and the palm leaves turning brittle.[265]

If you want to nurture bees in your garden, plant lemongrass. Lemongrass is also known as *gavati chaha* and is used in tea and in preparations for an herbal soup used to prevent coughs and colds. It is best known in Ayurvedic medicine to relieve the nasal congestion of a cold as well as coughs.[266]

The first samples of the closely-related citronella oil were displayed at the 1951 World's Fair in London's Crystal Palace. For hundreds of years in India it was known locally as *choomana poolu,* a reference to the plant's red grass stems. It is also reported that lemongrass was being distilled for export from the Philippines as early as the seventeenth century.[267]

Lemongrass is used as a smudge, like Native Americans use sage to purify spaces and drive off negative energies. The plant is dried, gathered into bundles, and burned. The smoke is the agent that purifies the air.

COMMON USES FOR LEMONGRASS ESSENTIAL OIL

- **Muscle relaxer:** mix 5 drops of lemongrass essential oil with 2 T of carrier oil and massage onto stiff muscles. (It works extremely quickly on a charley horse that can abruptly wake you in the middle of the night.)

---

264   "Lemongrass Health Benefits and Healing Properties | Ayurvedic Wellness & Lifestyle," planetwell.com.

265   Stella Temple, "Home of Pure Essential Oils," www.puressentialoils.co.za/newsletters .htm#Lemongrass.

266   "Lemongrass Health Benefits And Healing Properties | Ayurvedic Wellness & Lifestyle," planetwell.com.

267   "Lemongrass," www.herbalpedia.com/blog/?p=73.

- **Headache relief:** diffuse 4 drops of lemongrass essential oil for headache relief, or add 2 drops to a small bowl of warm water and soak a washcloth in the water. Wring out and apply to forehead as a compress. Repeat application until you feel relief. Place the washcloth on the back of your neck.

- **Depression lift:** diffuse a few drops of lemongrass essential oil daily.

- **Arthritis joint pain:** mix 4 drops of lemongrass essential oil and 1 drop of lavender essential oil into 2 T of carrier oil and rub onto affected and painful areas.

- **Shock:** if someone is in shock, add 1 or 2 drops of lemongrass essential oil to a cotton ball and place the infused cotton ball under the nostrils, not touching the skin. Do this right away and summon medical help.

- **For wound cleansing:** blend a few drops of lemongrass essential oil with witch hazel or a saline solution to flush wounds.

- **Heartburn aid:** mix 3 drops of lemongrass essential oil with a carrier oil and massage around the throat and chest area to relieve heartburn.

- **Indigestion:** a drop or 2 massaged into the abdomen, clockwise, will assist digestion and relieve the symptoms of indigestion.

- **To reduce a fever:** mix 10 drops of lemongrass essential oil with 1 T carrier oil in a roller ball applicator and apply to the back of neck, chest area, and the bottoms of your feet. This same blend works for insomnia. Rub diluted mixture onto feet at night.

- **To repel insects:** apply a few drops of lemongrass essential oil to the edges of your clothing to repel insects like ticks. If you apply to skin, be sure to dilute in a carrier oil before using.

- **Acne:** lemongrass essential oil is antimicrobial as well as a mild astringent. For acne relief add 1 drop lemongrass essential oil to 5 drops carrier oil and dab on to affected areas once or twice a day.

- **Oily skin:** place a drop of lemongrass essential oil in 8 oz. warm water and use as an astringent skin rinse.

- **Stress relief:** diffuse 5 to 6 drops of lemongrass essential oil or put a diluted drop on your palms, rub them together, and inhale the scent. You can also put a drop or 2 on a cloth or inside a pillowcase for stress relief while you sleep.

- **Fatigue relief:** diffuse 3 to 4 drops of lemongrass essential oil or mix a drop or 2 with 1 tsp. of carrier oil and massage into your temples.

- **High blood pressure:** lemongrass essential oil is a vasodilator and can help reduce high blood pressure by relaxing the blood vessels. Diffuse a few drops.

- **Fabulous hair:** mix 2 drops of lemongrass essential oil, 2 drops rosemary essential oil, and 1 drop of ginger essential oil into 1 oz. of your shampoo and use on your hair.

- **General pain relief:** mix 10 drops of lemongrass essential oil and 5 drops of clove bud essential oil with 2 tsp. carrier oil and pour into a 10 ml roller ball applicator. Shake well before each use then apply generously. Massage the area gently for quicker relief.

Cautions

Lemongrass essential oil should be avoided in pregnancy. Lemongrass essential oil can also irritate sensitive skin. Patch test before using. Avoid using if you have hypoglycemia.[268]

Lemongrass essential oil may be an alternative for individuals who are sensitive to peppermint essential oil. Tisserand and Young recommend a dermal maximum of .7 percent.[269]

---

268   "Pharmacognostical Investigation of Cymbopogon citratus (DC) Stapf" in *Der Pharmacia Lettre*, 2 (2) 2010, 181–189 via www.scholarsresearchlibrary.com.

269   Tisserand and Young, *Essential Oil Safety*, 334–335.

Blends Well With

Basil, bergamot, black pepper, cedarwood, clary sage, geranium, ginger, pink grapefruit, lavender, lemon, marjoram, orange, patchouli, rosemary, tea tree, thyme, vetiver, and ylang-ylang essential oils.

Supernatural Uses

Lemongrass is a major ingredient in the celebrated New Orleans-style van van oil, which is used to dress amulets.

Here's a spell adapted from Herbal Riot for landing a dream job: [270]
Find paper, a pen, lemongrass essential oil, your résumè, a fireproof plate, and a match or lighter. (Make sure you abide by safety precautions for an open flame indoors and out.)

1. On a new moon day, get a copy of your résumè and write long, detailed information about your dream job on the reverse side. Describe the dream job and imagine your feelings when you have landed it.

2. Place 1 drop lemongrass essential oil on the reverse side of the résumè.

3. Now fold the résumè in half and then in half again, continuing to fold a total of six times.

4. Place the folded résumè in a fireproof vessel and while seated near it, light the paper on fire. (Take great caution with this step and use a wind-free, fireproofed environment and receptacle.)

5. While it burns, visualize your life after you get the job. Extinguish all burned parts, douse with water, and dispose responsibly.

---

270   Crystal Aneira, "Get Me a Job Spell," herbalriot.tumblr.com/post/58418289002/the-magickal-uses-of-lemongrass.

34: Palo Santo

Loosely translated, palo santo means "holy wood" or "sacred wood." It has been used for hundreds of years by indigenous tribes shamans for spiritual applications.[271] It was used by the Incas to purify and cleanse the spirit from negative energies.[272] The aroma of palo santo is uniquely sweet and woody.

Its name originates from:

Latin: *Bursera graveolens*	**French:** *Palo santo*
Spanish: *Palo santo*	**English:** *Palo santo*
Gender: *Masculine*	**Ruling Planet:** *Sun*
Element: *Fire*	

Property Description

Anticancerous,[273] antiblastic,[274] anti-inflammatory, antibacterial, antifungal.

Benefits

Palo santo essential oil benefits include relieving symptoms of common colds, coughs, stress, headaches, anxiety, inflammation, emotional trauma, and more. It has qualities that help the regrowth of knee cartilage, reduce arthritis pain and inflammation, rheumatism, gout, respiratory problems, and reduce airborne contaminant when diffused. It has cancer-fighting properties, is a stimulant for the immune system, and supports a healthy nervous system.[275]

---

271 "Palo Santo Oil," www.aromaweb.com/essential-oils/palo-santo-oil.asp.

272 Ruby Gibson, *My Body, My Earth: The Practice of Somatic Archaeology* (Bloomington, IN: iUniverse, 2008), 83.

273 "Sacred Palo Santo Health Benefits," www.sacredpalosanto.com/benefits/.

274 Inhibits the growth of parasites.

275 Josh Axe, MD "Palo Santo Boosts Immune Health and Fights Inflammation," draxe.com /palo-santo/accessed 7/16/2015.

Palo santo helps support the immune system by turning off inflammatory responses created by a poor diet, pollution, stress, and illness.

Palo santo essential oil is widely used in folk medicine for stomachaches, as a sudorific, and as liniment for rheumatism. In one published Cuban medical study, components in the essential oil inhibited the growth of a specific type of breast cancer, MCF-7.[276]

Both palo santo and frankincense essential oils are used for emotional and spiritual support because they work as natural anxiety remedies.

After inhalation, palo santo travels directly through the olfactory system to the brain, where it helps to turn on the body's relaxation response to reduce panic, anxiety, and insomnia.[277] Palo santo can be used as a substitute for frankincense and myrrh in many blends.

In typing this section I misspelled "palo santo" a couple of times as "palo santa." Upon reflection, I think "palo santa" might not be a bad name for it because of all the gifts it brings.

Background

In Ecuador it is against the law to remove or cut down palo santo trees because they are protected. Additionally, even taking a dead tree has strong permit requirements by the government. Very few companies have permits to even touch the trees, let alone to produce palo santo essential oil.

The wood of the palo santo tree is of no earthly use unless the tree has died of natural causes. If a palo santo tree is cut into while it is still alive, it will need to undergo at least three years of a natural alchemical process of breaking down and decaying before it releases its precious oil. Native cultures believe that there are magical qualities to the tree and the spirits within materialize themselves as the oil. This is why the properties are believed to be healing and powerful.

Palo santo essential oil is distilled from the heartwood of the palo santo tree. The heartwood must be at least two years old and be from the red wood to produce the higher quality oil. The longer the tree has been dead, the more powerful the oil. This also holds true for frankincense essential oil.

---

276 Chris Kilham, "Palo Santo: A Frangrant Wood with Cancer Fighting Properties," www.foxnews.com/health/2013/10/02/palo-santo-fragrant-wood-with-cancer-fighting-properties/.

277 Christina Priano-Carrion, "Palo Santo: A Sacred and Spiritual Scent," thearomablog.com/a-sacred-and-spiritual-scent-palo-santo/.

There is a wonderful story shared by internationally certified Aromatherapist Cristina Proano-Carrion on her blog. According to legend, long before the world was born, a young lad named Crosokait was one of the very few humans alive. He fell in love with a young maiden but the love was unrequited. He fell ill with the sadness of rejection and although he called for her many times on his deathbed, she did not come. He uttered these dying words:

I'll always be with her, I will decorate her head with perfumed flowers. I will frighten insects away from her. I will give fragrance to the water that her lips drink. I will go to heaven in the aromatic smoke during the ceremony. I will be wherever she is and will give her whatever she asks for…

A tree grew up on the very spot where he was buried. When it was burned the wood released a deep, sweet aroma. The local Tobas tribe named it the palo santo tree as a symbol of love, kindness, and longing for an impossible love.[278]

Palo santo is used in South America in much the same way as white ceremonial sage is used in North America: to combat negative energy and to cleanse a space. Amazonian shamans use it in sacred plant spirit ceremonies; the rising smoke of the lit sticks is believed to enter the energy field of ritual participants to clear misfortune, negative thoughts, and chase away evil spirits.[279]

The Criollo people used the smoke of palo santo along with the burning leaves of *Ruta chalepensis* for patients with ear infections. *Ruta chalepensis* is commonly known as "fringed rue," a perennial herb native to Eurasia and North Africa, which has been traditionally used as an herbal remedy for inflammation and fever.

Palo santo's properties are also known to have been valued medicinally, by inhaling its smoke along with burning yerba mate leaves and even feathers of the rhea bird, (a flightless bird similar to an ostrich), for its healing effects.[280]

---

278   Christina Priano-Carrion, "Palo Santo: A Sacred and Spiritual Scent," thearomablog
.com/a-sacred-and-spiritual-scent-palo-santo/.

279   "Palo Santo Essential Herb," www.mountainroseherbs.com/products/palo-santo-essential
-oil/profile.

280   M. Nieves, "Metaphysical Properties of Holy Wood," www.gyvai.com/palo-santo-wood
-metaphysical-properties/.

Some protected palo santo comes from sustainably cultivated wood grown on a fifty-acre farm in Ecuador that contains both naturally occurring and replanted palo santo. To date they have replanted more than five thousand palo santo trees on the land to ensure an adequate supply for the future.

For those who use essential oils for meditation practice, prayer, or other spiritual applications, palo santo is an essential oil with exceptional merits.

COMMON USES FOR PALO SANTO ESSENTIAL OIL

- **Grounding:** mix 4 drops of palo santo essential oil with 5 drops cedarwood, 1 drop of patchouli, and 3 drops of bergamot essential oils. Use this blend in 2 T of carrier oil for massage or diffuse it.

- **Mind lifting:** mix 4 drops palo santo essential oil, 5 drops cedarwood essential oil, 1 drop patchouli essential oil, 5 drops of bergamot essential oil. Stir well. Diffuse or use mixed in 2 T carrier oil for a massage blend.

- **Meditation blend:** diffuse 3 drops of palo santo essential oil, 6 drops of lavender essential oil, 1 drop melissa essential oil, and 6 drops of frankincense essential oil. This blend will lift you to a higher vibration. As you inhale the scent feel it lifting your spirit, separating you from the worries of the day and taking you into a calm space.

- **Anti-anxiety bath:** mix into ¼ C Epsom salt, 4 drops of palo santo essential oil, 4 drops of lavender essential oil, and 2 drops of neroli essential oil. Add this mix to your bath water and allow the calming qualities to provide you with strength and comfort.

- **Pain relief:** mix 5 drops of palo santo essential oil, 5 drops of Roman chamomile essential oil, and 5 drops of grapefruit essential oil into 1 oz. of a carrier oil such as jojoba or sweet almond. Apply to the affected parts of your body.

- **Headache:** diffuse or inhale with eyes closed over steam a few drops of palo santo essential oil to relieve migraines, stress-related headaches, or bad moods.

- **For cold or flu relief:** apply a few drops of diluted palo santo essential oil on the chest at heart level or add some to your shower or bath to help arrest a cold or flu.

Cautions

Palo santo essential oil has been graded as nontoxic, nonirritant with possible skin sensitivity in some individuals. Do a patch test before applying directly to your skin.

Do not use during pregnancy. Tisserand and Young advise a dermal maximum of 3.4 percent.[281]

Blends Well With

Black pepper, cedarwood, clary sage, frankincense, lemongrass, myrrh, rose, sandalwood, and vetiver essential oils.

Supernatural Uses

Protection, remove negative energy, spiritual uplift, and purification.

Palo santo essential oil is used in ceremonial rituals, for vibrational work, and for clearing negativity.[282]

- Place a few drops of palo santo essential oil on a 1" piece of cloth to carry with you to attract good luck, repel negative energies, and communicate better with the spirits.

- Use a few drops diffused while setting and sealing your intentions or while cleansing your crystals and jewelry.

- **For emotionally charged issues:** diffuse palo santo essential oil for its grounding sense of peacefulness and calm. Use it to repel negative spirits.

- Diffuse a drop or 2 of palo santo essential oil for anxiety, emotional trauma, and depression.

---

281   Tisserand and Young, *Essential Oil Safety*, 379.

282   "Ceremonial," www.forheavensake.com/shop/category/ceremonial/.

- Diffuse or inhale palo santo essential oil to raise your vibration and to invite in a deeper connection to the earth and your divine source. Helps communicate with the spirit world.

- **For insomnia:** before bed, apply a couple of drops of diluted palo santo essential oil to the palm of your hands. Rub your hands together and close your eyes. Inhale deeply. Visualize being rooted and nourished by the earth. Experience the feeling of stability and strength. When you open your eyes, massage the soles of your feet with palo santo essential oil.

- Use palo santo essential oil as many times as you need to relax and reconnect with your higher consciousness. It lifts and purifies.

35: Pink Grapefruit

The grapefruit was known as the shaddock, shaddick, or shattuck until the nineteenth century. Botanically, it was not distinguished from the pomelo until the 1830s, when it was given the name *Citrus paradisi*. The grapefruit is thought to be the product of crossing an orange with a pomelo. Its true origins were not determined until the 1940s.

Its name originates from:

Latin: *Citrus paradisi*	**French:** *Pamplemousse*
Spanish: *Toronja*	**English:** *Grapefruit*
Gender: *Masculine*	**Ruling Planet:** *Sun*
Element: *Fire*	

Property Description

Antidepressant, antiseptic, aperitif, diuretic, disinfectant, lymphatic stimulant, tonic, anti-infectious, metabolic stimulant, detoxifier.

Benefits

Pink grapefruit essential oil, similar to other citrus fruit essential oils, has an elevating and relaxing effect on the mind.

In healthy adults, inhaled grapefruit oil was stimulating and invigorating, increasing the activity of the sympathetic nervous system by 50 percent, and causing a slight increase in skin temperature and slightly increased epinephrine and norepinephrine levels. [283]

It is said to ease muscle fatigue and stiffness. Pink grapefruit essential oil is sometimes added to creams and lotions as a natural toner and cellulite treatment. Like other citrus oils, it can ease nervous exhaustion and relieve depression.

Many have used grapefruit essential oil successfully for weight management. Using it daily can help decrease the appetite which leads to weight loss.

The diuretic properties of grapefruit essential oil promote urination and help in the removal of excess water, fats, sodium, uric acid, and other toxins from the body while also reducing blood pressure for a healthy heart. [284]

Background

One story of the fruit's origins is that Captain Shaddock brought "palmelo" seeds to Jamaica from Indo-China in the 1640s and grew the first fruit. [285] The name shifted to "pamelo" and then to "shaddock." Rev. Griffith Hughes wrote about grapefruit in the 1759 *Natural History of Barbados*:

> **Forbidden-Fruit-Tree:** The Trunk, Leaves, and Flowers of this Tree, very much resemble those of the Orange-tree. The Fruit, when ripe, is something longer and larger than the largest Orange; and exceeds, in the Delicacy of its Taste, the Fruit of every Tree in this or any of our neighboring Islands.

---

283   S. Haze, K. Sakai, and Y. Gozu, "Effects of Fragrance Inhalation on Sympathetic Activity in Normal Adults." *The Japanese Journal of Pharmacology* 90(3), 2002, 247–253.

284   "Herbal Oil: Grapefuit Essential Oil Benefits and Uses," healthyss.com/health-benefits -of-grapefruit-essential-oil/2/.

285   J. Kumamoto, R. W. Scora, H. W. Lawton, and W. A. Clary, "Mystery of the forbidden fruit: Historical epilogue on the origin of the grapefruit, Citrus paradisi," *New York Botanic Garden*, www.jstor.org/pss/4254944.

It hath somewhat of the Taste of a Shaddock; but far exceeds that, as well as the best Orange, in its delicious Taste and Flavor.[286]

The grapefruit was brought to Florida as seeds by Spanish nobleman Don Phillippe, who migrated to Florida in 1808, bringing with him the new and improved shaddock. Initially, he gave many cuttings and trees away to anyone who wanted them and an eager Captain A. L. Duncan accepted some of those first seedlings. Duncan rapidly became a successful, prominent grower of grapefruit among other citrus varieties. He perfected growing techniques, such as grafting, with the help of the US Department of Agriculture and produced a fine specimen known as the Duncan grapefruit.

Along came Kimball Chase Atwood, a pioneer, visionary, and wealthy entrepreneur, who also became enamored of the grapefruit and founded the Atwood Grapefruit Company in the late nineteenth century specifically to corner the market on growing and shipping worldwide. Pink grapefruit was first discovered in 1906 at his orchards appropriately named the Atwood Grove in Florida.[287]

The differences between the white and pink grapefruits are minor and only a matter of production. Pink grapefruit is sweeter than the white variety and is therefore more in demand. The therapeutic values are identical.

Common Uses for Pink Grapefruit Essential Oil

- **Wake-me-up:** keep pink grapefruit essential oil by your bedside. On those morning when it is difficult to get up, place a few diluted drops in your hands, rub together, inhale, and you'll have the spring in your step needed to get up and get going. The same technique works as a pick-me-up during the day.

- **Self-esteem:** inhale a few drops of diluted pink grapefruit essential oil either from your hands or over a steaming pot of water. Add 5 drops of

---

286 Other essential oils that also repel mosquitos and can be included in the blend are: cedarwood, tea tree, geranium, rosemary, lemongrass, citronella, and eucalyptus essential oils.

287 Charles Atwood, "1978 Atwood Grapefruit Company," www.manateecountyhistoricalsociety .com/1978–atwood-grapefruit-company/.

pink grapefruit essential oil to steaming water, cover your head with a towel, close your eyes and inhale for 4 to 5 minutes. After inhalation, you may feel a renewed sense of empowerment.

- **Shiny hair:** adding 1 to 2 drops of pink grapefruit essential oil to your shampoo bottle will result in a lustrous shine. Pink grapefruit essential oil has also been shown to help reduce oily scalp and other skin and hair conditions.[288]

- **Body refresher:** mix 4 drops of pink grapefruit essential oil with 2 T of carrier oil and massage clockwise onto your torso to stimulate the lymphatic system, liver, and gallbladder.

- **Room freshener:** diffuse 4 to 5 drops of pink grapefruit essential oil to disinfect and freshen a room.

- **For weight loss/appetite and craving suppressant:**

  1. Place 1 or 2 drops of diluted pink grapefruit essential oil into the palms of your hands. Rub together then cup your hands and inhale the fragrance for 5 minutes three times a day.

  2. Breathe in the scent of diffused pink grapefruit 5 to 20 minutes prior to a meal. Drink 8 oz. of pure water after inhaling the oil. You can alternate this technique with peppermint essential oil or black pepper essential oil or both for appetite suppression.

  3. Add 1 or 2 drops of patchouli essential oil to 3 drops of pink grapefruit essential oil and inhale per the above instructions. Patchouli essential oil enhances the benefits of the pink grapefruit essential oil and can be a natural appetite suppressant.

- Pink grapefruit essential oil can help to diminish appetite but it also can assist a sluggish digestion and increase metabolism.

---

288 Jo Hartley, "Amazing Benefits of Pink Grapefruit Essential Oil," www.naturalnews .com/030838_pink_grapefruit_health_benefits.html.

- **Hangover:** in case of over-indulgence, use a steam inhalation technique to restore your electrolyte balance by adding 4 to 5 drops of pink grapefruit oil and 2 drops of basil essential oil to a basin of steaming water and cover your head with a towel and close your eyes. Lean over the basin to inhale the fumes. After about 5 minutes you should begin to feel the relief from too much partying, depending, of course, on how much partying was done.

- **Relieve oily skin:** add a few drops of pink grapefruit essential oil to your face creams and lotions to help unclog pores and refresh skin.

Cautions

Any grapefruit essential oil may have negative interactions with statin drugs, medications that are used to help lower cholesterol. Do not use if you are taking statins. Consult your doctor first.

Grapefruit oil is listed as nontoxic, nonirritant, nonsensitizing. It is listed as phototoxic and may cause the skin to react if exposed to strong sunlight after topical treatment. Wait 12 to 24 hours before going out in the sun after use. Do not use if oil has oxidized. Dermal maximum of .4 percent to avoid phototoxic reactions.[289]

Blends Well With

Geranium, lavender, black pepper, bergamot, clary sage, clove bud, eucalyptus, frankincense, ginger, lemon, neroli, patchouli, peppermint, thyme, rosemary, and ylang-ylang essential oils.

Supernatural Uses

Protection, healing, opens crown chakra to your higher purpose.

- **Increase optimism:** inhale or diffuse a few drops of pink grapefruit essential oil to remove blocked thinking and hopeless resignation.

- **Recapture your childhood free spirit:** inhale or diffuse a few drops of pink grapefruit essential oil. (The urge to skip down the street may invade your feet.)

---

289 Tisserand and Young, *Essential Oil Safety*, 297.

- Inhale or diffuse a few drops of pink grapefruit essential oil to become more stable and aligned with your higher self and guiding inner mind.

- Anoint an icon or an amulet with a drop of pink grapefruit essential oil for protection. Wear it around your neck in a pendant diffuser or keep on your person in a sacred pouch. If it touches your body, make sure the oil is diluted.

- Meditation is enhanced by diffusing a few drops of pink grapefruit essential oil and visualizing your crown chakra opening.

- Place 1 or 2 drops pink grapefruit essential oil on a 1" piece of cloth and carry with you for healing of your emotions and self-worth.

36: Dill

Dill (*Anethum graveolens*) is generally thought to have its beginnings around the Mediterranean region. The Latin name is a combination of the words *ano* and *theo*, which together mean "upward I run."[290]

Anethum also originates from the Greek word *aneson* or *aneton*, which is most likely also the origin of the name "anise."[291]

The Latin name *graveolens* comes from a combination of two words; *gravis*, meaning heavy or weighty, and *oleo*, which means "producing a smell or odor." When combined into *graveolens* the meaning of these two words becomes "emitting a heavy odor."[292]

I like to think of dill as having the spiritual meaning of moving forward and smelling great.

---

290 Arthur O. Tucker, PhD, and Thomas DeBaggio, *The Big Book of Herbs: A Comprehensive Illustrated Reference to Herbs of Flavor and Fragrance* (Ft. Collins, CO: Loveland Publishing, 2000).

291 Gernot Katzer, "Anise," gernot-katzers-spice-pages.com/engl/Pimp_ani.html.

292 Amanda Formano, "The Herb Society of America's Guide to Dill," www.herbsociety.org /herbs/documents/Dillguidenewer.pdf.

Its name originates from:

Latin: *Anethum Graveolens*	**French:** *Aneth*
Spanish: *Eneldo*	**English:** *Dill, aneton,*
Gender: *Masculine*	*dilly, dill weed, chebit,*
Element: *Fire*	*sowa, keper, hulwa*
	Ruling Planet: *Mercury*

Property Description

Antispasmodic, anti-inflammatory, digestive, carminative, stomachic, disinfectant, sedative.

Benefits

The health benefits of dill essential oil include its ability to boost digestive health as well as provide relief from insomnia, hiccups, diarrhea, dysentery, menstrual disorders, respiratory disorders, and cancer. It is also used for oral care (bad breath).

It can be a powerful boost for the immune system and can also offer protection from bone degradation.[293]

Dill has been used for flavoring foods as well as for medicinal purposes. Both the seeds and the leaves are used. Dill exudes a strong, tangy, appetizing flavor. Dill contains compounds called monoterpenes, as well as flavonoids, minerals, and certain amino acids.[294]

Traditionally, dill-based herbal remedies were used in treating stomach disorders, to reduce intestinal gas, and to calm the digestive system.

Dill essential oil is still used as a remedy to relieve painful intestinal spasms, muscular cramps, and as an aid to alleviate colic in children.[295]

---

293   Susan Melgren, "7 Detox Herbs for a Natural Cleanse," www.motherearthliving.com /natural-health/7–detox-herbs-natural-cleanse.aspx.

294   "Dill," www.goenkaexim.com/dill.aspx.

295   "Dill," crookedbearcreekorganicherbsandflowers.wordpress.com/tag/dill/.

Background

The earliest known record of dill as a medicinal herb was found in Egypt five thousand years ago when the plant was referred to as a soothing medicine.[296] Dill was also popular among Greeks and Romans, too.

Dill was commonly regarded as the Anethon of Dioscorides. It was well known in Pliny's days and was often mentioned by writers in the Middle Ages. As a drug it has been used by healers since ancient times. It is even mentioned in the tenth-century vocabulary of Alfric, Archbishop of Canterbury.[297]

The name "dill" is derived, according to *Prior's Popular Names of English Plants*, from the Old Norse word, *dylla* (to lull) referring to the carminative properties of the drug.[298]

Dill seeds were historically nicknamed "meetinghouse seeds" because they were chewed during long church services to keep members awake, quiet the children, freshen bad breath, and quiet noisy stomachs.

Dill is native to southern Russia, western Africa, and the Mediterranean region. It is a hardy annual that grows wild among the corn in Spain and Portugal and along the coastal regions of Italy.

Dill was mentioned both in the Bible and in ancient Egyptian writings. It was popular in the ancient Greek and Roman cultures, where it was considered a sign of wealth and was revered for its many healing properties.

Dill was used by Hippocrates, the father of medicine, in a recipe for cleaning the mouth.[299]

Ancient soldiers would apply roasted dill seeds to their wounds to promote healing. In ancient Roman times, gladiators were fed meals covered with dill because it was hoped that the herb would grant them valor and courage.[300]

---

296 "The Herb Society of America's Essential Facts for Dill," www.herbsociety.org/documents /DillAnethumgraveolens.pdf.

297 E. A. Weiss, *Spice Crops* (Wallingford, UK: CABI Publishing, 2002), 279.

298 Maude Grieve, "Dill," www.botanical.com/botanical/mgmh/d/dill—13.html.

299 "World's Healthiest Foods," www.whfoods.com/genpage.php?tname=foodspice &dbid=71.

300 Stella Mira, "Spicy Challenge," www.dokuga.com/forum/29—challenges/86683—spicy -challenge.

Charlemagne even made it available on his banquet tables, so his guests who indulged too much could benefit from its carminative (gas releasing) properties. Today, dill is a highly noted herb in the foods of Scandinavia, central Europe, North Africa, and Russia.[301]

COMMON USES FOR DILL ESSENTIAL OIL

- **For weight control:** place 2 drops of diluted dill essential oil into the palms of your hands and rub together. Cup your hands and take several deep whiffs of the oil. Do this for several minutes about 20 minutes prior to meals. You can also use this technique when you crave sweets or a snack during the day. Alternate sessions with pink grapefruit essential oil.

- **Skin repair:** mix a few drops of dill essential oil into your face cream or lotion. It will help clear up skin and heal wounds.

- **For restful sleep:** blend 3 drops of dill essential oil with 3 drops of cedarwood essential oil into 1 T carrier oil and massage into neck and shoulders. Or, diffuse same blend without the carrier oil 30 minutes before bedtime.

- **Stress reliever:** diffuse 3 drops of dill essential oil with 1 drop bergamot essential oil and 1 drop lemon essential oil to lessen anxious feelings.

- **Detox:** massage 1 or 2 drops of dill essential oil diluted in a carrier oil into the soles of your feet to support detoxification. (You can also create a roller ball applicator using 5 drops of dill essential oil and 1 tsp. carrier oil and roll that onto your soles and alternate with other essential oils to avoid sensitization.)

- **Calming:** diffuse 3 drops of dill essential oil as needed, or inhale 1 drop diluted dill essential oil and 1 drop diluted Roman chamomile essential oil rubbed between your hands. Do this for at least a full minute. Repeat if needed.

---

301 "World's Healthies Foods," www.whfoods.com/genpage.php?tname=foodspice&dbid=71.

Cautions

Do not use dill essential oil if pregnant or breastfeeding.

The most common side effect of dill oil is skin irritation, especially for people who are allergic to plants that belong to the carrot family. Dermal maximum recommended is 1.4 percent.[302]

Blends Well With

Lemon, orange, and other citrus oils as well as bergamot, clove bud, vetiver, lemongrass, and helichrysum essential oils.

Supernatural Uses

Offers protection from black magic, brings happiness, good fortune, blessings.

- Take a bath infused with 3 or 4 drops of dill essential oil bath to become irresistible. Disperse oil in almond, coconut, or rice milk.

- Add 1 or 2 drops of dill essential oil to a 1" piece of cloth. Place it under your pillow to become tantalizing to your lover.

- Add 2 drops of dill essential oil to curtains in children's rooms to protect them from evil spirits and guard them against bad dreams. (Pre-test for staining.)

- Purchase a charm, icon, or a symbol for your front door. Anoint it with dill essential oil so that no one unfriendly or envious of you can enter your house.

- Use diluted dill essential oil as the curator of the breath of life. Dill essential oil supplies the courage to look at the sources of our painful emotions.

- Use dill essential oil on a vision quest to foster inner wisdom.

- Anoint a charm or talisman with dill essential oil to provide protection from spells. Carry with you or wear on your person.

---

302   Tisserand and Young, *Essential Oil Safety*, 269.

- Add dill essential oil to love potions and aphrodisiacs to increase their effectiveness.

- In a small pouch, place a quarter. Add some drops of dill essential oil and carry with you to attract money. (Use a higher bill denomination if you prefer.)

Honorable Mentions

There are so many wonderful, top-quality essential oils available. It was a difficult and challenging process of elimination to pare my selections down to just thirty-six in these three palettes of tools for the healing artist.

Not all oils could be included in this book, and you'll probably discover more on your own that become your favorites. In fairness to the honorable mentions, the following paragraphs detail some of the rationale I would like to share with you about a few essential oils that were neck and neck with the top thirty-six that were chosen.

Bay laurel essential oil, *Laurus nobilis,* is very close in therapeutic value to ravensara and benzoin essential oils. It helps relieve colds, virus infections, mouth ulcers, the respiratory system, muscle aches and pains, arthritis, sinus headache, and is an insect repellent. There is another essential oil called bay but this is not the same family as bay laurel or ravensara essential oils.

Cypress essential oil, *Cupressus sempervirens,* is distilled from wood. Earlier we chose cedarwood essential oil and palo santo essential oil for our list. All three are members of the *Cupressaceae* botanical family. I like cypress essential oil for its historical and sacred uses, but we already have its therapeutic qualities in the other essential oils from the same family.

Elemi essential oil, *Canarium luzonicum,* is in the same family, *Burseraceae,* as benzoin, palo santo, myrrh, and frankincense essential oils. Elemi essential oil is good for skin care including wrinkles and skin tone. We have the benefits of elemi essential oil covered with the above relatives plus lavender and helichrysum essential oils.

Juniper berry essential oil, *Juniperus communis.* Cedarwood covers many of the therapeutic values that juniper berry essential oil has. It can assist colds, flu, acne, cellulitis, gout, hemorrhoids, obesity, rheumatism, and toxic build-up. Acne is helped by tea tree, lavender, clary sage, and rose essential oils. Colds and flu symptoms are quelled by peppermint, eucalyptus, and lemon essential oils. Rheumatism is aided by tea tree, lemon, frankincense, and myrrh essential oils. Obesity and weight control are helped by ginger, black pepper, pink grapefruit, and dill essential oils.

Nutmeg essential oil, *Myristica fragrans,* comes from the *Myristicaceae* family. Its properties have anti-fungal and anti-microbial properties that fight against *Streptococcus mutans.* Our other anti-fungals are tea tree, myrrh, cedarwood, and eucalyptus essential oils. Our anti-bacterial/anti-microbial essential oils are cinnamon, melissa, clove bud, and ravensara. Clove was one of the herbs found in the blend from the four thieves who escaped the fifteenth-century plagues in Europe by dousing themselves with aromatic infused herbal vinegars.

Oregano essential oil, *Oreganum vulgare,* is from the *Labiate* family possessing anti-viral, anti-fungal, and anti-parasitic therapeutic qualities. It is a spectacular essential oil, but we have the benefits covered with rosemary and peppermint essential oils which are close relatives and do the same job. Oregano is not used frequently in aromatherapy, but you might come across it and wonder if you should use it or not, hence this notation.

Pine essential oil, *Pinus sylvestris,* is an anti-fungal and anti-microbial essential oil. Its smell is divine and refreshing, but it can be a bit overwhelming especially if you grew up in a household that used Pine Sol for cleaning. Having the same therapeutic qualities as pine essential oil are: tea tree, ravensara, thyme, lavender, patchouli, helichrysum, and peppermint essential oils.

Spearmint essential oil, *Mentha spicata/Mentha cardiac,* is very close to peppermint essential oil and is part of the *Labiatae* mint family of wonderful healers. Having similar benefits to spearmint essential oil are: lavender, rosemary, melissa, and marjoram essential oils.

Add any other essential oils you wish to your collection. Owning all of them is nothing short of a cornucopia of riches. The top thirty-six I recommend are just a beginning as there are more than three hundred essential oils in the marketplace for you to choose from. Just remember to make sure you buy organic, identify their properties and benefits and use them with love and respect, and follow the cautions.

TEN

The Master's Palette: 14 Premium Essential Oils and Absolutes

It's my hope that you have already taken the plunge and are loving your essential oils. Have you noticed any changes in your life because of them? I can only live vicariously through you and imagine that you are relishing them and letting your creative genius experiment with the gorgeous oils. So much information all at once can be a bit overwhelming. I hope that you have enjoyed reading about each essential oil, taken the learning process one step at a time, and been patient and thrilled with your unfolding journey.

Every time I take my precious essential oils out of their case I get excited all over again. I use them for myself, I make inhalers and blends for my friends and clients, and I experiment with new concoctions all of the time. Nothing feels better to me than watching someone's life improve because they have used one of the blends I created especially for them. I wish I could share what you are doing with your essential oils and watch how you are using them. I enjoy seeing the results of what truly creative minds design.

The upcoming master's palette of essential oils contains a list of all of the essential oils and absolutes I dream about owning and using. I've purchased *samples* and small sizes of most of them over the years and consider them a super treat for special occasions. As you are able, please treat yourself to some of the essential oils and absolutes on the list below. I think you'll find them quite incredible.

The master's palette contains a list of some of the most amazing-smelling essential oils and absolutes in the world. Many are used by the perfume industry. The reasons for the high prices are their extraordinary fragrance, their healing properties, and the fact that it requires an enormous amount of products/blossoms to make one ounce of essential oil. For your convenience, I have arranged them in order of the most expensive.

1. Champaca, *Michelia champaca* — $2,250 USD oz.
2. Tuberose, *Polianthes tuberosa* — 1,650 USD oz.
3. Coffee flower, *Coffea canephora* — 1,600 USD oz.
4. Frangipani, *Plumeria alba* — 1,500 USD oz.
5. Cannabis flower, *Cannabis sativa* — 950 USD oz.
6. Agarwood, *Aquilaria agallocha* — 850 USD oz.
7. Rose bulgarian, *Rosa x damascena* — 800 USD oz.
8. Seaweed, *Fucus vesiculosus* — 650 USD oz.
9. Elencampe, *Inula helenium* — 560 USD oz.
10. Sandalwood (Indian), *Santalum album* — 450 USD oz.
11. Carnation, *Dianthus carophyllus* — 425 USD oz.
12. Jasmine, *Jasminum officinale* — 250 USD oz.
13. Blue chamomile, *Matricaria recutita* — 180 USD oz.
14. Hops, *Humulus lupulus* — 160 USD oz.

Below are some further descriptions about each of these premium essential oils and absolutes.

1: Champaca

Champaka (also a correct spelling) is considered most precious among the Indian flowers. It is a southern Asian tree, *Michelia champaca,* from the *Magnoliaceae* family, having fragrant yellow or orange flowers and yielding champaca essential oil, which is used in perfumes. It is also referred to as golden champaca, and possesses a delightful aroma that is a rich, sensual, full-bodied blend of exotic florals with a spicy apricot undertone. *Michelia champaca* is native to the lowlands of central India (also growing in Nepal, Malaysia, Indonesia, and the Philippines). It is a small evergreen tree that bears a multitude of lemon-yellow flowers, the source of the essential oil.

Champaca has been used to treat the blues for centuries. Indians traditionally use this essential oil/absolute to cure headaches and vertigo.

Its name originates from:

Michelia champaca/Nag champa **Absolute**	
Latin: *Michelia champaca* **Plant source:** *Flowers* **Origin:** *India*	**English:** *Champaca, champaka, champak, golden champaca, champak sapu, champa, champaca flower*

Benefits
Relaxing, euphoric effects, similar to the benefits of jasmine or neroli essential oils.

Common Uses
Perfume blends, calming aromatherapy diffusion, mood-lifting, and spiritual.

Blends Well With
Carnation, jasmine, neroli, orange, rose, sandalwood, and ylang-ylang essential oils.

Cautions
Check for skin sensitivity using a skin patch test before using topically.

2: Tuberose

Tuberose, *Polianthes tuberosa*, is very popular and highly valued among perfume manufacturers. Its flower has a beautiful fragrance, which is solely active at night, meaning this is the only time when this mysterious nocturnal flower blooms.

Tuberose is often called "night queen" or "mistress of the night." It grows well in Central America and India and is in high demand in the perfume trade. I remember one incredible afternoon when I was a guest at an elegant hacienda in Colima, Mexico. We were invited to horseback ride around the base of the Colima volcano through the acres and fields of flowering tuberose.

The fragrance in the air was not of this world. In an instant I was part of the ethereal world. I will never forget how that felt.

Its name originates from:

Polianthes tuberosa Absolute	
Latin: *Polianthes tuberosa* **Plant source:** *Flowers*	**Origin:** *India* **English:** *Tuberose, night queen, mistress of the night*

Benefits
Aphrodisiac, deodorant, relaxing, sedative, and warming substance. Anti-inflammatory and antioxidant.

Common Uses
Tuberose essential oil is used in perfume blends, is diffused as a calming agent, has been used to repel mosquitos, is a trusted mood enhancer and effective aphrodisiac.

Blends Well With
Bergamot, clary sage, frankincense, geranium, lavender, neroli, orange, patchouli, rose, sandalwood, carnation, coffee flower, and vetiver essential oils.

Cautions
Requires a patch test for skin sensitivity. Dermal maximum of 1.2 percent.[303]

---

303   Tisserand and Young, *Essential Oil Safety*, 456–457.

3: Coffee Flower

This essential oil is beyond dreamy. It comes from the coffee plants grown wild and in the forests of Madagascar and on farms. It is as rare as it is incredible.

Coffee and wood farming have devastated the rain forests of Madagascar since 1950. Only half of the original forest remains so it is crucial to buy this essential oil from companies that support sustainable and organic farming.

Madagascar grows both arabica and robusta coffee plants. The flowers that make up our essential oil come from the c. robusta plant. The plant looks like a small tree, flowers only in September, and each blossom is harvested individually by hand.

Harvesting traditionally begins at sunrise and only the blossoms that are just beginning to unfold are selected.

Flowers that have already opened quickly wither and lose their oils shortly after picking. Unopened buds continue to produce their precious volatile oils even after gathering.

Distillation must occur immediately in order to preserve the essence and aroma of the coffee flower bud oil. Solvent extraction is the method used for efficiently extracting the fragrant molecules of the plant.

Its name originates from:

Coffea canephora **Essential Oil**	
Latin: *Coffea canephora*	**Origin:** *Madagascar*
Plant source: *Flowers and buds*	**English:** *Robusta coffee*

Benefits

Purifying, transformative, uplifting, spiritual, balancing, opens the heart, brings joy and pleasure. An important part of this essential oil is that the flowers of this robusta plant require cross pollination to bloom and this activity creates the sense of yin-yang balance the arabica plant does not have.

Common Uses

Skin conditioner, hair enhancer, massage oil, calms the nervous system, reduces anxiety, and exudes peace and comfort.

Blends Well With

Bergamot, cinnamon, ginger, melissa, tuberose, neroli, orange, rose, carnation, sandalwood, and ylang-ylang essential oils.

Cautions

Before using on skin be sure to do a patch test. Dilute before diffusing as this is a powerful essence.

4: Frangipani

Frangipani essential oil, *Plumeria alba*, is intensely floral with a musk note scent including a back note of hay and honey. They have an intoxicating fragrance that is positively transportive when inhaled.

Frangipani (plumeria) is the most fragrant and desirable of all flowers for Hawaiian leis. The frangipani is the national tree of Laos, where it is called *dok jampa* and considered to be sacred. Every Buddhist temple in that country has planted frangipani bushes in their courtyard. Many of the trees are hundreds of years old and are visually spectacular as huge, gnarly giants.

In India the frangipani is a symbol of immortality because of its ability to produce leaves and flowers even after it has been lifted out of the soil. Like in Laos, it is often planted near temples and graveyards, where the fresh flowers fall daily on the burial tombs.[304]

In Caribbean cultures the leaves are used as poultices (a healing wrap) for bruises and ulcers and the latex (sap) is used as a liniment for rheumatism.[305]

---

304   "About Frangipanis" www.allthingsfrangipani.com/frangipanis.html.
305   Ibid.

Its name originates from:

Plumeria Essential Oil	
Latin: *Plumeria alba*	**Origin:** *France*
Plant source: *Flowers*	**English:** *Plumeria, frangipani, temple flower, may flower*

Benefits

Aphrodisiac, restores peace and harmony, calming, sedative, astringent, anti-inflammatory, antioxidant, air purifier.

Common Uses

Hair conditioner, skin soother and moisturizer, inflammation reduction, love spells.

Blends Well With

Bergamot, clary sage, clove bud, ginger, pink grapefruit, lemon, neroli, orange, patchouli, rose, carnation, coffee flower, sandalwood, and ylang-ylang essential oils.

Cautions

Avoid in pregnancy and on babies and children.

5: Cannabis Flower

Cannabis flower essential oil has many powers and healing properties. It is often sold as hemp essential oil but should not be confused with hemp seed essential oil. The cannabis flower essential oil we are referring to contains no THC (delta-9–tetrahydrocannabinol) that is found in marijuana. It is an unusual oil because it comes from the same plant source as marijuana but is not used for any purposes other than healing.

Originally used two thousand years ago in India, Persia, and the Middle East, cannabis flower essential oil was used in religious ceremonies and burial rituals. It was associated with the Norse goddess Freya and handed down to the Celts after the Viking invasions.

It is used in soups, perfumes, soaps, candles, and other goods. It requires fifty pounds of flower buds to render an ounce of oil. Because it is a powerful essential oil, only small amounts are required for healing.

Blogger Jeff Callahan, creator of EssentialOilBenefits.org, clarifies the legal situation and benefits of cannabis flower essential oil:

> Despite the illegal status of cannabis in many parts, serious research is increasingly showing that use of cannabis flower essential oil has the potential to fight cancer, multiple sclerosis, rheumatoid arthritis, Alzheimer's disease and Lou Gehrig's disease.[306]

Its name originates from:

Latin: *Cannabis sativa, Cannabis indica* **Plant source:** *Flowers and upper leaves*	**Origin:** *India, Middle East* **English:** *Cannabis flower, hemp flower, hemp blossom, cannabis blossom*

Benefits
Antioxidant, anti-inflammatory, sedative, antifungal, antiallergenic.

Common Uses
Cannabis flower essential oil has been used to reduce stress and anxiety, relieve depression and insomnia, regulate cardiovascular function, rejuvenate skin, decrease eczema and arthritis pain, and stimulate eye health for better vision and abate macular degeneration.

Blends Well With
Spicy and citrusy oils, vetiver, and patchouli.

---

306   Jeff Callahan "Cannabis Flower Essential Oil," essentialoilbenefits.org/cannabis-flower
      -essential-oil/.

Cautions

There are no outstanding contraindications for the use of this essential oil. If you are taking medications, get permission from your doctor before using this oil. There may be legal restrictions in your area.

Although it is an extremely gentle oil, it is very powerful so it should be used sparingly, with caution and diluted.

6: Agarwood

The scent of agarwood is complex and quite pleasing. Agarwood essential oil was historically prominent having great cultural and religious significance in ancient civilizations. It was mentioned in one of the world's oldest written texts, the Sanskrit Vedas from India.

In China as early as the third century CE the chronicle *Nan Zhou Yi Wu Zhi* ("Strange Things From the South") written by Wa Zhen of the Eastern Wu Dynasty mentioned agarwood as being produced in central Vietnam. He described in detail how people collected it in the mountains.

Agarwood's use as a medicinal product has been recorded in the *Sahih Muslim*, a collection of hadith from the prophet Mohammed, dating back to approximately the eighth century, and in the Ayurvedic *Susruta Samhita* medicinal text.[307]

Famous for its sensual undertones, agarwood has been known for centuries as an aphrodisiac. It has also been featured as key incense for spiritual prayer rituals because of its strong biblical ties to Adam and Eve. (It is believed by some texts that Adam covered his nakedness with the leaves from the agarwood tree.)

Agarwood essential oil is by far one of the most precious and expensive essential oils. Each tree may take more than three hundred years to produce resin, which makes agarwood essential oil very rare. It has a woody, nutty, deep, honey, earthy, mossy, balsamic, bittersweet aroma. The scent of a single drop will last for hours.

---

307 Edward Bouverie Pusey, *Daniel the Prophet: Nine Lectures, Delivered in the Divinity School of the University of Oxford* (New York: Funk & Wagnalls, 1885).

"Today, the demand for agarwood far exceeds supply. A recent study revealed that supply rates are only 40 percent of the demand and a liter of agarwood oil can be sold for around $10,000–$14,000 USD on the market (Vietnam Chemical Technology Institute, 2007). Indeed agarwood is reputed to be the most expensive wood in the world and it is estimated that specialized buyers are prepared to pay as much as ten times more for this product." [308]

Its name originates from:

Aquilaria agallocha Essential Oil	
Latin: *Aquilaria agallocha*	**Origin:** *Assam, India*
Plant source: *Wood*	**English:** *Oud, oohd, ouhd, aloeswood, agarwood*

Benefits

Improves symptoms of depression. Helps induce relaxation. Improves lung/respiratory conditions.

Common Uses

Can be used as a perfume, applied topically diluted, in a warm compress, in a bath, inhaled, or diffused.

Blends Well With

Rose absolute, rose otto, frankincense, sandalwood, myrrh, geranium, carnation, and neroli essential oils.

Cautions

It is nontoxic, nonsensitizing, and nonirritant. Be sure to do a patch test before using on your skin in case of sensitivity.

---

308 Joachim Gratzfeld and Bian Tan, "Agarwood—saving a precious and threatened resource," www.bgci.org/resources/article/0576/.

7: Bulgarian Rose

Organic Bulgarian rose (*Rosa x damascena*) is expensive because gathering the flowers must be done by hand, making the process quite labor intensive. There are only twenty to forty days per year when harvesting occurs, depending on the type of *Rosa damascena*, cultivated in the region. The roses are gathered individually and carefully brought to a central location for steam distillation.

Historians believe that the cultivation of the Kazanlak rose, *Rosa x damascena* began in 1420 and is grown in the Valley of the Roses near Kazanlak in Bulgaria. Supposedly a Turkish judge around the fifteenth century brought roses from Tunisia and cultivated them in his own fragrant garden.[309]

Its name originates from:

Rosa x damascena **Absolute** or **Otto**

Benefits

Rose essential oil is one of the best antidotes for people with stress and anxiety. It harmonizes the spirit, enhances performance of the brain and soothes the nervous system to reduce the effects of stress. Refer to chapter 8, number 14 for the details about rose essential oil.

8: Seaweed

Seaweed is a general nomenclature used for the more than nine thousand varities of species of algae and marine plants that breed in various water bodies like rivers and oceans. Seaweeds grow in a wide range of sizes from minuscule to gigantic. Most seaweed is medium-sized and available in multiple colors like red, brown, and green.

Its name originates from:

Fucus vesiculosus **Absolute**

---

309 "Rose Otto," aromanation.com/rose_otto.html.

Benefits

Seaweed absolute benefits cancer, obesity, diabetes, influenza, and radiation poisoning. It helps by improving digestion, teeth, the cardiovascular system, and helps to maintain healthy skin and hair. Seaweed contains cancer-fighting agents that may prove useful in curing tumors and other cancer conditions like colon cancer and leukemia.[310]

In the ocean, seaweed plays an extremely vital role for marine life. It is a foundation for the majority of food chains and is home for many marine creatures. Seaweed contains anti-microbial and anti-inflammatory properties that have provided health benefits to humans since ancient times.

Seaweed absolute's anti-inflammatory properties have shown relief for people suffering with osteoporosis and rheumatoid arthritis. Seaweed absolute also has properties that aid in enriched blood circulation and boosting the immune system.

Chinese Medicine doctors have used hot water extracts of certain seaweeds in the treatment of cancer. Both Japanese and Chinese medicine have used seaweeds to treat goiter and other glandular problems since 300 BCE.[311]

The Romans used seaweeds in the treatment of wounds, burns, and rashes. The Celts noted that ordinary seaweed contracted as it dried and then expanded with moisture. In Scotland during the eighteenth century, physicians used dried seaweed stem to successfully drain abdominal wall abscesses.[312]

Common Uses

Marine-inspired perfumes, arthritis relief.

Blends Well With

Grapefruit, lemon, lime, ylang-ylang, geranium.

---

310   "Health Benefits of Seaweed," www.organicfacts.net/health-benefits/other/health-benefits
-of-seaweeds.html.

311   "Seaweed" www.drugs.com/npp/seaweed.html.

312   Ibid.

Cautions

People taking aspirin or any medicinal blood thinner might be affected due to the blood-thinning effect of seaweed. This is a thick, viscous oil. Dilutes well in jojoba oil.

9: Elecampane

Elecampane has been known for centuries as a valuable herbal medicine. It produces yellow flowers and is native to Europe. Originally it was used as a treatment for horses and sheep but research in the 1800s showed its value for humans.[313]

The herb is most successfully harvested in the autumn. It has a somewhat bitter, herbal, sweet floral taste, but the early Romans enjoyed it as an herbal stomachic and used it in a digestive wine known as *potio paulina*.[314]

Its name originates from:

Elecampane **Essential oil**	
Latin: *Inula helenium* **Plant source:** *Root and flowers* **Origin:** *Southern and Eastern Europe*	**English:** *Elencampe, scabwort, elf dock, wild sunflower, horseheal, velvet dock, yellow starwort*

Benefits

Antispasmodic, analgesic, cholagogue, diuretic, diaphoretic, expectorant, stimulant, astringent, carminative, antiseptic, stomachic, emmenagogue.

Common Uses

Digestive, food additive, chest infections, cough relief.

Blends Well With

Sage, peppermint, lavender, hops, and thyme essential oils.

---

313 "Elecampane," essentialoilbenefits.org/elecampane-essential-oil.

314 Ibid.

Cautions

Excessive use can trigger diarrhea, allergies, and nausea. It should not be used by pregnant women.

You will need guidance and some experienced training before using this essence. It can have contraindications for diabetes and blood sugar levels.

10: Indian Sandalwood

Please refer to chapter 7, number 10 for more about sandalwood essential oil.

Its name originates from:

Santalum album **Essential Oil**

Benefits

Sandalwood essential oil has been used for two thousand years and is one of the most recognized fragrances in the world. Chinese Medicine uses it for healing and it is popularly combined with rose to produce the famous Indian scent, *aytar*.

Because of limited resources, sandalwood essential oil has now become quite expensive. Due to strict restrictions imposed from over-harvesting the source, the original Indian sandalwood is no longer readily available in the consumer market. The majority comes from Australia. As sustainable ecology increases, you may be able to find some genuine Indian sandalwood essential oil that is government sanctioned. This substance needs to be researched and carefully purchased from sustainable growers and harvesters.

11: Carnation

The carnation was cultivated by the Greeks and Romans to use in ceremonial crowns. The name *carnis* comes from the Latin word meaning "flesh." Some Christians believe it was the flower of the incarnation when God was made flesh. The formal name for carnation, *dianthus*, comes from the Greek botanist Theophrastus who called it the "heavenly flower."

The flower has come down through the ages being something symbolic. It is the official flower of Mother's Day in the US and red carnations are associated with love, pink with gratitude, and green with St. Patrick's Day. It is also the national flower of Spain.

Carnation aromas have been used by artists, writers, and poets to induce a state of inspirational euphoria and to stimulate creativity and productivity. Carnation teas were used in ancient Chine to promote energy, vitality, and stimulate ch'i.

Its name originates from:

Dianthus carophyllus **Absolute**	
Latin: *Dianthus carophyllus*	**Origin:** *Mediterranean area, China*
Plant source: *Flowers*	**English:** *Carnation, clove pink*

Benefits
Antiseptic, styptic, sedative, antidepressant, antianxiety.

Common Uses
Muscle spasms, promoting energy and vitality, soothing the body, and bringing peace to the soul.

Blends Well With
Jasmine, rose, grapefruit, lavender, carnation, patchouli, and ylang-ylang essential oils.

Cautions
Floral oils require a patch test to ensure safety and no adverse skin reaction.

12: Jasmine

Like frangipani, jasmine (*Jasminum officinale*) is also known as "Queen of the Night." For hundreds of years it has been a favorite fragrance for women. Pure jasmine essential oil can be very expensive because the delicate blossoms are carefully collected before sunrise to prevent the fragrance from evaporating. Jasmine essential oil has been used throughout history for assisting romance and attraction.

Its name originates from:

Jasminum officinale Essential Oil/Absolute	
Latin: *Jasminum officinale* **Plant source:** *Flowers*	**Origin:** *Asia, Africa, Australasia* **English:** *Royal jasmine, Spanish jasmine, Catalonian jasmine, jati*

Benefits

Jasmine essential oil/absolute soothes, relaxes, uplifts, and enhances self-confidence. It is helpful for the skin and popular in skin care products due to its balancing nature. Jasmine essential oil has been found to reduce anxiety, stress and depression. It has also been used to improve wrinkles, eczema, and greasy skin.[315]

Common Uses

The essential oil can also be inhaled directly or diffused undiluted. Use it mixed into your face cream for skin enhancement. Diffuse it to balance emotions and reduce stress.

Blends Well With

Bergamot, clary sage, frankincense, geranium, orange, carnation, lavender, neroli, rose, and sandalwood essential oils.

Cautions

Dilute jasmine essential oil in a carrier oil before applying to skin. Tisserand and Young recommend a dermal maximum of .7 percent.[316]

---

315 "Aromatherapy for Education, Entertainment and Well-Being," khealing.com /blogbeautyasweage.html.

316 Tisserand and Young, *Essential Oil Safety*, 311–313.

13: Blue Chamomile

Chamomile essential oils come in two versions. We have selected Roman chamomile essential oil as one of the primary palette essential oils. Blue or German chamomile essential oil is another great oil and could be another wonderful choice for your essential oil collection.

Blue chamomile is native to Europe and northern Asia. It is cultivated in Hungary, France, Eastern Europe, and Egypt.[317]

Blue chamomile essential oil is extracted from *Matricaria recutita*, or *Chamomilla recutita* of the same family, and is also known by the names of Hungarian chamomile and single chamomile. Blue chamomile essential oil has a sweet, straw-like fragrance and is dark blue in color.

Its name originates from:

Matricaria chamomilla Essential Oil	
Latin: *Matricaria recutita, or Chamomilla recutita*	**English:** *German chamomile, single chamomile, Hungarian chamomile*
Plant source: *Flowers*	**Other Names:** *Baboonig, babuna, babuna camornile, babunj*
Origin: *Egypt*	

Benefits

Analgesic, antiallergenic, antispasmodic, antibiotic, anti-inflammatory, antiphlogistic, bactericidal, carminative, cicatrisant, cholagogue, emenagogue, hepatic, digestive, sedative, stomachic, vermifuge, vasoconstrictor, and vulnerary.

Blue chamomile essential oil is generally safe for use in adults and children. It relieves pain, and helps skin heal from burns, eczema, rashes, and inflammatory conditions. Inhaling blue chamomile essential oil lowers stress and helps to counteract allergies and insomnia, leading factors in anxiety.

Blue chamomile essential oil is extracted from tiny daisy-like flowers and contains a beautiful blue volatile oil (azulene).

---

317   "German Chamomile," materiaaromatica.com/Default.aspx?go=ProductDisplay
&ProductID=25485.

Common Uses

Blue chamomile essential oil has a calming effect on the mind and body, is excellent in treating any type of inflammation, and is very effective on urinary stones (bladder gravel) as well.[318] It is good for acne, arthritis, bruises, congestion, cramps, cuts, digestion, emotional healing, hair, skin, and sleep.

For skin issues, it is a miracle worker that calms red, dry, irritated skin, as well as calming allergies, eczema, psoriasis, and all other flaky-type skin problems.

Blends Well With

Bergamot, clary sage, orange, geranium, lavender, rose, carnation, hops, sandalwood, and ylang-ylang essential oils.

Cautions

Chamomile is one of the safest herbs around but some people can be allergic to this plant or any member of the ragweed family.

Check for sensitivity by doing a patch test of the essential oil to a small area of the skin. Also check with your doctor before using as it may have interactions with some drugs.

14: Hops

Very similar to barley, hops originates in southeast Asia as well as China, and it has been used to flavor and ferment beer for more than ten thousand years. Hops are currently grown across the northern hemisphere from England to the US and Canada.

Its name originates from:

Humulus lupulus **Essential Oil**	
Latin: *Humulus lupulus, related to cannabis*	**Origin:** *China, England, Germany, Canada, United States*
Plant source: *Flowers*	**English:** *Hops*

---

318   "German Chamomile," www.aromashop.in/chamomile-essential-oil.

Benefits

Sedative, calmative, anti-inflammatory, anti-viral, analgesic, anti-spasmodic, stomachic.

Common Uses

Hops essential oil has a sedative nature and can bring relief from respiratory conditions by reducing the inflammation and irritation in the lungs and bronchial passages.

It can calm the spasms of coughs; alleviate headaches; improve skin rashes, psoriasis, and eczema; aid indigestion, insomnia, and dandruff; add gloss and shine to hair,; and reduce or alleviate menstrual cramps.[319] Although hops are used in the brewing and fermentation of beer products, hops essential oil is also helpful for those needing help quelling their desire for alcohol. For this purpose, the most effective use of hops essential oil is in a diffuser.

Blends Well With

Cinnamon, ginger, nutmeg, pine, balsam, pink grapefruit, lemon, and orange essential oils.

Cautions

If you suffer from severe depression, it is recommended that you do not use this oil due to its sedative qualities. Use only under the supervision of a qualified Aromatherapist. Also, certain types of skin may react to this potent oil, so use it with a high dilution of carrier oil and do a patch test before applying to skin. Skin reactions have been recorded with improper use.

Hops essential oil is potent. Be sure you monitor your exposure to it when used in a diffuser or mixed with a carrier oil. Pre-testing your response to the oil is essential and smart. Hops essential oil can also reduce libido, so make sure you plan ahead before using this oil.

---

319   James Bowe, Xiao Feng Li, James Kinsey-Jones, Arne Heyerick, Susan Brian, Stuart Milligan, Kevin O'Byrne. "The Hop Phytoestrogen, 8–prenylnaringenin, Reverses the Ovariectomy-induced Rise in Skin Temperature in an Animal Model of Menopausal Hot Flashes," www .ncbi.nlm.nih.gov/pmc/articles/PMC1635969/.

PART THREE

Additional Uses

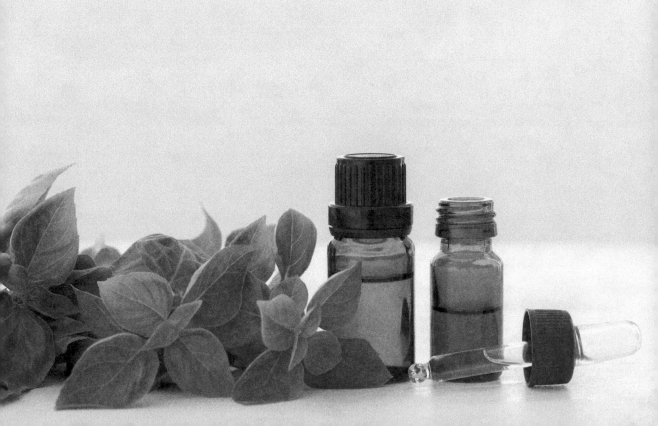

ELEVEN

Essential Oils for Assisting Emotions

Emotions are dynamic, constant conversations between the body and the mind. The Dalai Lama calls them bridges. Emotions are active, living impulses and they can affect the mind/brain and be affected by the mind/brain in return. The pathway is reciprocal. When we are attempting to heal our bodies, emotions, or minds, we can tap into our feelings and intentionally change our emotions to serve our purpose. Essential oils help us focus on our issues—our blockages—alleviate them, and move into a better life.

For example, if we are constantly living in a state of panic, urgency, or frustration, we stimulate hormones in our bodies that produce cortisol and lead to many diseases ranging from heart plaque to weight gain, diabetes, and high blood pressure. If we use essential oils that target relaxation, forgiveness, balance, harmony, and weight control, we'll turn our lives around.

If we suffer from low self-esteem, don't believe in ourselves, or are constantly self-critical, we may be prone to suffer from depression, failure, procrastination, addiction to drugs or alcohol, weight gain, and a suppressed immune system, which leaves us vulnerable to illness. We can use essential oils that allow us to forgive ourselves, release the past, re-energize, achieve mental clarity, and begin to feel good about ourselves. We can turn our negative spiral into positive action.

If we are confused in life or in the middle of a huge transition and in need of spiritual and emotional support, essential oils can provide that for us, too.

Human vibrational frequencies can be raised through the sensory mechanism of the limbic system (smell brain) using essential oils; we might be wise to put them to effective use.[320]

Essential oils can, according to research, effect changes in the emotions which translate into changes in the body. Choosing a specific oil to create the emotional shift we desire is one of the many benefits of using essential oils for personal improvement.

Emotions wake us up and make us pay attention to what's going on in the world around us. Paying attention may very well be the key to healing. Not only is it a matter of defense but when we pay attention to what is happening or not happening in our bodies and environment, we stay more in tune with our personal world and well-being. We also can protect ourselves from harm using this level of awareness.

Many spiritual teachers call this *mindfulness*. Essential oils are tools which allow us to use mindfulness to stay steady in the rocky sea of life. They are true bridges of change between the mind and the body.

Emotions are complex experiences and there are many facets to consider when dealing with them. Each living person has a different emotional signature. My emotional needs may not be your emotional needs and we may respond dissimilarly to a remedy or solution. You may have a fear of flying; I may not.

I may have an aversion to spiders; you may keep them as pets. We can either embrace our feelings and live with them, or we can use essential oils to harness our emotional responses and shift them to better serve our lives and purposes.

You can begin by using the following categories as guidelines for your emotional healing work. Experiment. Be sure to sniff each essential oil and allow your physical and sentient reaction to determine whether a particular oil is right for you or not.

You can also muscle test (kinesiology) the individual essential oils and gauge if they are a match for your bodily chemistry. Video instruction for muscle testing is available on the Internet and on YouTube.

Below are some essential oil possibilities for working with your emotions. They are categorized by emotion with suggestions for essential oils that can help manage and

---

320 "The Smell Report," www.sirc.org/publik/smell_emotion.html.

change certain feelings. Cross-check the individual descriptions of the essential oils in this book by name to see why they are listed as a specific remedy.

Anger: Basil, Roman chamomile, bergamot, geranium, melissa, marjoram, neroli, orange, patchouli, rose, sandalwood, vetiver, ylang-ylang

Anxiety: Basil, lavender, Roman chamomile, neroli, bergamot, cedarwood, clary sage, frankincense, marjoram, palo santo, patchouli, spikenard, tea tree, ylang-ylang

Clarity (mental): Cedarwood, rosemary, lemon, basil, peppermint, geranium, clary sage, tea tree

Confidence-boosting: Bergamot, pink grapefruit, frankincense, orange, cedarwood, lemongrass, melissa, rose, sandalwood ginger, rosemary, ylang-ylang

Confusion (eliminating): Tea tree, lemon, rosemary, peppermint, basil, black pepper, orange

Courage: Black pepper, ginger, thyme, yarrow, frankincense, dill, thyme, spikenard, helichrysum

Decision-making: Ylang-ylang, frankincense, clove bud, geranium, peppermint, lemon, pink grapefruit, sandalwood, rosemary

Depression: Bergamot, clary sage, rose (if depression is due to grief), frankincense, geranium, pink grapefruit, helichrysum, jasmine, lavender, spikenard, Roman chamomile, ylang-ylang, neroli, lemon, orange, sandalwood

Fatigue (burnout): Basil, bergamot, clary sage, cypress, eucalyptus, frankincense, ginger, pink grapefruit, helichrysum, lemon, marjoram, melissa, patchouli, peppermint, thyme, rosemary, sandalwood, vetiver

Fear: Bergamot, cedarwood, frankincense, ginger, pink grapefruit, neroli, orange, Roman chamomile, sandalwood, spikenard, vetiver, lavender, geranium, marjoram

Fear of the future: Dill, frankincense, ylang-ylang, melissa, lavender, palo santo, sandalwood, spikenard

Forgiveness: Frankincense, rose, myrrh, spikenard, bergamot, geranium, lemon, melissa, ylang-ylang

General emotional stress: Melissa, geranium, sandalwood, bergamot, vetiver, rose, clary sage, black pepper, ginger, marjoram, basil, neroli, orange, frankincense

Gratitude: Frankincense, myrrh, geranium, ylang-ylang, ginger, orange, neroli, pink grapefruit, bergamot

Grief: Rose, melissa, frankincense, helichrysum, neroli, palo santo, sandalwood, vetiver

Grounding: Basil, frankincense, lavender, Roman chamomile, rose, geranium, jasmine, marjoram, ylang-ylang, sandalwood, cedarwood, palo santo, patchouli, vetiver

Happiness: Bergamot, cedarwood, geranium, pink grapefruit, lemon, melissa, helichrysum, neroli, orange, palo santo, sandalwood, ylang-ylang, rose, frankincense

Heart (broken/closed/wounded): Rose (full concentration), rosemary, basil, neroli, helichrysum, black pepper, palo santo, ylang-ylang, patchouli, peppermint

Insecurity: Bergamot, cedarwood, frankincense, jasmine, sandalwood, rose, vetiver, ylang-ylang

Inner child work (drawing out/befriending): Bergamot, orange, neroli, sandalwood, jasmine, lemongrass, ylang-ylang

Insomnia: Clary sage, dill, lavender, lemongrass, marjoram, neroli, palo santo, spikenard, clove bud, yarrow, geranium, bergamot, Roman chamomile

Irritation: Lavender, neroli, roman chamomile, orange, sandalwood, patchouli, spikenard

Jealousy: Rose, Roman chamomile, palo santo, vetiver, ylang-ylang

Joy: Neroli, orange, bergamot, lavender, lemon, melissa, pink grapefruit, helichrysum

Lethargy: Rosemary, black pepper, peppermint, dill, ginger, clove bud

Loneliness: Bergamot, clary sage, frankincense, helichrysum, orange, frankincense, palo santo, Roman chamomile, rose

Memory (Improvement): Lemon, melissa, thyme, rosemary, peppermint, basil, black pepper, pink grapefruit, lavender, clary sage, sandalwood

Panic: Roman chamomile, ylang-ylang, rose, frankincense, lavender, neroli, helichrysum

Peace: Roman chamomile, frankincense, lavender, bergamot, palo santo, sandalwood, ylang-ylang, rose, pink grapefruit, lemon, geranium

Strength: Myrrh, palo santo, dill, melissa, cedarwood, lemon

Self-confidence: Bergamot, clary sage, sandalwood, jasmine, pink grapefruit, melissa, rose, myrrh, frankincense, orange, patchouli, rosemary, ylang-ylang

Stress reduction: Bergamot, clary sage, frankincense, geranium, pink grapefruit, jasmine, lavender, lemon, neroli, palo santo, patchouli, Roman chamomile, rose, ravensara, sandalwood, vetiver, ylang-ylang

Workaholism: Geranium, lavender, basil, bergamot, melissa, neroli, marjoram

Following are some basic recipes that you may want to begin with. I've taken suggestions from Aromatherapists around the world and devised what are the most pleasing recipes for me and my clients. That said, nothing is engraved in stone—find the blends and combinations that work best for you.

The absolute joy and satisfaction is experimenting with your own blends until you find the right one that resonates with you on every level of your mind, body, and spirit. You can muscle-test the blends to see how your body responds at the subconscious level. The body never lies. It will show you if a blend is healing and right for you or not. All you have to do is pay attention and listen to your body.

These suggested blends are meant only as a beginning. You know yourself, your preferences, and your needs better than anyone else, so you can be as creative as you want to be and become your own personal essential oil chef.

As you excel with blending, try different combinations of the essential oils listed next to each emotion. Add into your blend only the oils that resonate with your sense of smell. Sniff each one. Give it a moment to settle into your brain. Make a decision as to whether that one is *good* for you. If you react positively to it, place a few drops in the blend. Start with the undiluted essential oils first. Observe how they comingle, then ask, "Do they require something more?"

If you want to diffuse them, you can use a portion of the blend undiluted by carrier oils. Most diffusers function best with just the essential oils. Some brands can handle blending the essential oils with carrier oils. Read the instructions carefully to see what your diffuser manufacturer suggests and follow those guidelines. My diffuser can handle a blending so I like to add a few drops of a carrier oil to the diffuser blends because I find it mixes into the blend and creates a smooth commingling of the oils. Your diffuser may clog if you mix in carrier oils.

If you want to use a specific blend as a massage oil be sure to dilute it with a carrier oil. (Sweet almond, apricot kernel, or jojoba work nicely.) In chapter six you read about the general proportions for essential oil massage blends and diffuser proportions. In chapter fourteen you will learn about inhaler-making, roller ball applicator use, and some face and body cream recipes containing essential oils. Here are my suggestions for blends that are effective with various emotional states.

Anger Management Blends
One:
1–2 oz. carrier oil
1 drop rose essential oil
3 drops orange essential oil
1 drop palo santo essential oil
1 drop vetiver essential oil
Use as a massage oil blend

Two:

1 oz. carrier oil

2 drops Roman chamomile essential oil

2 drops ylang-ylang essential oil

1 drop orange essential oil

1 drop rose essential oil

Use as a massage oil blend

ANXIETY BLEND

One:

1 oz. carrier oil

2 drops bergamot essential oil

2 drops clary sage essential oil

1 drop frankincense essential oil

1 drop melissa essential oil

1 drop ravensara essential oil

Use as a massage oil blend

Two:

1 oz. carrier oil

1 drop patchouli essential oil

2 drops lavender essential oil

1 drop vetiver essential oil

1 drop sandalwood essential oil

2 drops orange or neroli essential oil

Use as a massage oil blend

For Diffuser:

9 drops lavender essential oil

6 drops clary sage essential oil

2 drops ravensara essential oil

4 to 6 drops carrier oil

CLARITY (MENTAL) BLEND

One:

1 oz. carrier oil

1 drop basil essential oil

3 drops rosemary essential oil

2 drops clary sage essential oil

1 drop peppermint essential oil

Use as a massage oil blend

Two:

1 oz. carrier oil

2 drops peppermint essential oil

2 drops lemon essential oil

1 drop orange essential oil

1 drop tea tree essential oil

Use as a massage oil blend

For Diffuser:

2 drops rosemary essential oil

1 drop basil essential oil

1 drop clary sage essential oil

1 drop lemon essential oil

1 drop cedarwood essential oil

3 drops carrier oil

CONFIDENCE ENHANCEMENT BLEND

One:

1 oz. carrier oil

3 drops orange essential oil

2 drops rosemary essential oil

1 drop pink grapefruit essential oil

1 drop lemongrass essential oil

Use as a massage oil blend

Two:

1 oz. carrier oil

4 drops bergamot essential oil

1 drop ylang-ylang essential oil

Use as a massage oil blend

For Diffuser:

3 drops bergamot essential oil

2 drops ylang-ylang essential oil

3 drops carrier oil

Confusion (eliminating) Blend

One:

1 oz. carrier oil

1 drop peppermint essential oil

8 drops orange essential oil

6 drops basil essential oil

1 drop dill essential oil

Use as a massage oil blend

Two:

1 oz. carrier oil

2 drops black pepper essential oil

2 drops lemon essential oil

2 drops tea tree essential oil

Use as a massage oil blend

For Diffuser:

1 drop black pepper essential oil

1 drop lemon essential oil

2 drops basil essential oil

1 drop clove bud essential oil

1 drop frankincense essential oil

3 drops carrier oil if your diffuser can
handle a carrier oil without clogging

Courage Blend

One:

1 oz. carrier oil

2 drops black pepper essential oil

1 drop ginger essential oil

1 drop thyme essential oil

1 drop dill essential oil

1 drop eucalyptus essential oil

Use as a massage oil blend

Two:

2 drops ginger essential oil

2 drops thyme essential oil

1 drop black pepper essential oil

1 drop spikenard essential oil

Use as a massage oil blend

For Diffuser:

1 drop ginger essential oil

1 drop thyme essential oil

2 drops black pepper essential oil

2 drops spikenard essential oil

1 drop yarrow essential oil

3 drops of carrier oil

Decision-making Blend

One:

1 oz. of carrier oil.

3 drops rosemary essential oil

2 drops peppermint essential oil

2 drops lemon essential oil

1 drop clove bud essential oil

1 drop palo santo essential oil

Use as a massage oil blend

Two:

1 oz. carrier oil

2 drops ylang-ylang essential oil

2 drops pink grapefruit essential oil

1 drop rosemary essential oil

2 drops lemongrass essential oil

Use as a massage oil blend

For Diffuser:

2 drops sandalwood essential oil

2 drops rosemary essential oil

1 drop lemon essential oil

1 drop dill essential oil

3 drops carrier oil

Depression (lifting) Blend

One:

1 oz. carrier oil

2 drops frankincense essential oil

1 drop lemon essential oil

2 drops ylang-ylang essential oil

1 drop neroli essential oil

2 drops ravensara essential oil

Use as a massage oil blend

Two:

1 oz. carrier oil.

1 drop lavender essential oil

1 drop ylang-ylang essential oil

3 drops pink grapefruit essential oil

Use as a massage oil blend

For Diffuser:

2 drops lavender essential oil

1 drop ylang-ylang essential oil

1 drop neroli essential oil

1 drop frankincense essential oil

1 drop geranium essential oil

3 drops carrier oil

Fatigue Blend

One:

1 oz. carrier oil

2 drops basil essential oil

1 drop cypress essential oil

2 drops pink grapefruit essential oil

1 drop eucalyptus essential oil

Use as a massage oil blend

Two:

1 oz. carrier oil

2 drops peppermint essential oil

1 drop frankincense essential oil

3 drops lemon essential oil

1 drop sandalwood essential oil

Use as a massage oil blend

Three:

1–2 T of carrier oil

3 drops ylang-ylang essential oil

2 drops rose essential oil

2 drops bergamot essential oil

1 drop helichrysum essential oil

1 drop neroli essential oil

1 drop clary sage essential oil

1 drop vetiver essential oil

Use as a massage blend or diffuse without the carrier oil

For Diffuser:

2 drops peppermint essential oil

2 drops frankincense essential oil

1 drop patchouli essential oil

4 drops carrier oil if your diffuser can
    handle a carrier oil without clogging

FEAR BLEND

One:

1 oz. carrier oil

3 drops sandalwood essential oil

2 drops orange essential oil

1 drop spikenard essential oil

1 drop cedarwood essential oil

Use as a massage oil blend

Two:

1 oz. carrier oil

2 drops clary sage essential oil

2 drop Roman chamomile essential oil

1 drop vetiver essential oil

2 drops lavender essential oil

Use as a massage oil blend

For Diffuser:

2 drops vetiver essential oil

2 drops orange essential oil

1 drop lemongrass essential oil

3 drops carrier oil if your diffuser can
    handle a carrier oil without clogging

FEAR OF THE FUTURE BLEND

One:

1 oz. of carrier oil

2 drops lavender essential oil

2 drops ylang-ylang essential oil

1 drop frankincense essential oil

1 drop dill essential oil

Use as a massage oil blend

Two:

1 oz. carrier oil

2 drops ylang-ylang essential oil

1 drop sandalwood essential oil

1 drop lavender essential oil

Use as a massage oil blend

For Diffuser:

2 drops ylang-ylang essential oil

2 drops spikenard essential oil

2 drops benzoin essential oil

2 drops carrier oil if your diffuser can
   handle a carrier oil without clogging

Forgiveness Blend
One:

1 oz. carrier oil

2 drops rose essential oil

1 drop bergamot essential oil

1 drop lemon essential oil

1 drop melissa essential oil

Use as a massage oil blend

Two:

1 oz. carrier oil

2 drops lemon essential oil

2 drop ylang-ylang essential oil

1 drop rose essential oil

Use as a massage oil blend

For Diffuser:

2 drops lemon essential oil

2 drops bergamot essential oil

1 drop rose essential oil

3 drops carrier oil if your diffuser can
    handle a carrier oil without clogging

GENERAL ALL-OVER EMOTIONAL STRESS BLEND

One:

1 oz. carrier oil

3 drops bergamot essential oil

2 drops vetiver essential oil

2 drops rose essential oil

1 drop geranium essential oil

1 drop cinnamon essential oil

Use as a massage oil blend

Two:

1 oz. carrier oil

7 drops neroli essential oil

4 drops lavender essential oil

5 drops lemon essential oil

1 drop melissa essential oil

Use as a massage oil blend

For Diffuser:

3 drops rose essential oil

2 drops vetiver essential oil

2 drops bergamot essential oil

3 drops carrier oil if your diffuser can
    handle a carrier oil without clogging

GRATITUDE BLEND

One:

1 oz. carrier oil

6 drops bergamot essential oil

3 drops pink grapefruit essential oil

4 drops myrrh essential oil

4 drops frankincense essential oil

3 drops ylang-ylang essential oil

2 drops ginger essential oil

Use as a massage oil blend

Two:

3 drops pink grapefruit essential oil

1 drop ginger essential oil

3 drops ylang-ylang essential oil

2 drops frankincense essential oil

1 drop myrrh essential oil

Use as a massage oil blend

For Diffuser:

2 drops ylang-ylang essential oil

1 drop frankincense essential oil

1 drop ginger essential oil

1 drop pink grapefruit essential oil

3 drops carrier oil if your diffuser can
   handle a carrier oil without clogging

GRIEF (RECOVERY) BLEND

One:

1 oz. carrier oil

1 drop rose essential oil

1 drop helichrysum essential oil

1 drop palo santo essential oil

2 drops frankincense essential oil

1 drop melissa essential oil

Use as a massage oil blend

Two:

1 oz. carrier oil

2 drops rose essential oil

3 drops sandalwood or palo santo essential oil

Use as a massage oil blend

For Diffuser:

1 drop rose essential oil

2 drops helichrysum essential oil

1 drop frankincense essential oil

1 drop vetiver essential oil

3 drops carrier oil if your diffuser can
    handle a carrier oil without clogging

GROUNDING BLEND

One:

1 oz. of carrier oil

2 drops frankincense essential oil

2 drops sandalwood essential oil

1 drop rose essential oil

1 drop vetiver essential oil

2 drops lavender essential oil

Use as a massage oil blend

Two:

1 oz. carrier oil

2 drops vetiver essential oil

2 drops cedarwood essential oil

1 drop patchouli essential oil

1 drop geranium essential oil

Use as a massage oil blend

For Diffuser:

2 drops lavender essential oil

2 drops sandalwood essential oil

1 drop rose essential oil

1 drop cedarwood essential oil

2 drops carrier oil if your diffuser can
handle a carrier oil without clogging

Happiness Blend

One:

1 oz. carrier oil

1 drop geranium essential oil

2 drops frankincense essential oil

2 drops orange essential oil

1 drop melissa essential oil

1 drop rose essential oil

Use as a massage oil blend

Two:

1 oz. carrier oil

3 drops bergamot essential oil

2 drops ylang-ylang essential oil

1 drop pink grapefruit essential oil

1 drop lemon essential oil

Use as a massage oil blend

For Diffuser:

2 drops sandalwood essential oil

1 drop rose essential oil

2 drops bergamot essential oil

6 drops carrier oil

Heart (broken, closed) Blend

One:

1 oz. carrier oil

3 drops rose essential oil

1 drop basil essential oil

1 drop melissa essential oil

1 drop patchouli essential oil

1 drop helichrysum essential oil

Use as a massage oil blend

Two:

1 oz. carrier oil

2 drops rosemary essential oil

2 drops basil essential oil

1 drop peppermint essential oil

1 drop helichrysum essential oil

Use as a massage oil blend

For Diffuser:

2 drops rose essential oil

1 drop basil essential oil

1 drop helichrysum essential oil

3 drops carrier oil if your diffuser can
handle a carrier oil without clogging

Insecurity Blend

One:

1 oz. carrier oil

3 drops bergamot essential oil

1 drop frankincense essential oil

2 drops ylang-ylang essential oil

1 drop sandalwood essential oil

1 drop palo santo essential oil

Use as a massage oil blend

Two:

1 oz. carrier oil

2 drops cedarwood essential oil

1 drop sandalwood essential oil

1 drop vetiver essential oil

Use as a massage oil blend

For Diffuser:

3 drops bergamot essential oil

2 drops frankincense essential oil

2 drops ylang-ylang essential oil

3 drops carrier oil if your diffuser can
    handle a carrier oil without clogging

Inner Child Blend (when working with healing/ drawing out your inner child)

One:

1 oz. carrier oil

2 drops ylang-ylang essential oil

1 drop neroli essential oil

1 drop rose essential oil

1 drop lemongrass essential oil

Use as a massage oil blend

Two:

1 oz. carrier oil

2 drops neroli essential oil

1 drop lemongrass essential oil

1 drop ylang-ylang essential oil

1 drop orange essential oil

Use as a massage oil blend

For Diffuser:

2 drops orange essential oil

1 drop lemongrass essential oil

1 drop sandalwood essential oil

3 drops carrier oil if your diffuser can
handle a carrier oil without clogging

INSOMNIA BLEND

One:

10 drops Roman chamomile essential oil

5 drops clary sage essential oil

5 drops bergamot essential oil

*Add 1 or 2 drops of this blend to tissue or
cloth and place inside your pillow*

Two:

5 drops lavender essential oil

2 drops bergamot essential oil

1 drop Roman chamomile essential oil

*Add 1 or 2 drops of this blend to tissue and
place inside your pillow*

For a Diffuser:

2 drops Roman chamomile essential oil

1 drop clary sage essential oil

1 drop bergamot essential oil

2 drops lavender essential oil

2 drops carrier oil if your diffuser can handle
a carrier oil without clogging

For a roller ball applicator:

To 1 T carrier oil add:

20 drops lavender essential oil

1 drop spikenard essential oil

7 drops palo santo essential oil

Mix into roller bottle and roll onto feet
before bed each night

IRRITATION BLEND

One:

1 oz. carrier oil

2 drops neroli essential oil

4 drops sandalwood essential oil

2 drops yarrow essential oil

Use as a massage oil blend

Two:

1 oz. carrier oil

2 drops lavender essential oil

1 drop neroli essential oil

2 drops Roman chamomile essential oil

1 drop spikenard essential oil

Use as a massage oil blend

For Diffuser:

2 drops Roman chamomile essential oil

2 drops neroli essential oil

1 drop lavender essential oil

1 drop spikenard essential oil

2 drops carrier oil if your diffuser can
handle a carrier oil without clogging

JEALOUSY BLEND

One:

1 oz. carrier oil

2 drops rose essential oil

3 drops Roman chamomile essential oil

1 drop vetiver essential oil
Use as a massage oil blend

Two:
1 oz. carrier oil
3 drops lavender essential oil
1 drop rose essential oil
2 drops palo santo essential oil
2 drops Roman chamomile essential oil
Use as a massage oil blend

For Diffuser:
2 drops rose essential oil
2 drops lavender essential oil
1 drop vetiver essential oil
3 drops carrier oil

Joy Blend
One:
1 oz. carrier oil
2 drops bergamot essential oil
2 drops pink grapefruit essential oil
1 drop rose or neroli essential oil
1 drop melissa essential oil
Use as a massage oil blend

Two:
1 oz. carrier oil
1 drop pink grapefruit essential oil
2 drops orange essential oil
1 drop lemon essential oil
1 drop neroli essential oil
Use as a massage oil blend

For Diffuser:

2 drops bergamot essential oil

2 drops pink grapefruit essential oil

1 drop orange essential oil

4 drops carrier oil if your diffuser can
handle a carrier oil without clogging

Lethargy Blend

One:

1 oz. carrier oil

2 drops rosemary essential oil

1 drop black pepper essential oil

1 drop eucalyptus essential oil

2 drops ginger essential oil

1 drop clove bud essential oil

Use as a massage oil blend

Two:

1 oz. carrier oil

5 drops pink grapefruit essential oil

3 drops rosemary essential oil

2 drops lavender essential oil

1 drop dill essential oil

Use as a massage oil blend

For Diffuser:

3 drops pink grapefruit essential oil

2 drops rosemary essential oil

1 drop black pepper essential oil

3 drops carrier oil if your diffuser can
handle a carrier oil without clogging

LONELINESS BLEND

One:

1 oz. carrier oil

1 drop rose essential oil

2 drops frankincense essential oil

2 drops bergamot essential oil

1 drop clary sage essential oil

Use as a massage oil blend

Two:

1 oz. carrier oil

3 drops bergamot essential oil

2 drops Roman chamomile essential oil

Use as a massage oil blend

For Diffuser:

3 drops bergamot essential oil

1 drop helichrysum essential oil

1 drop Roman chamomile essential oil

1 drop palo santo essential oil

3 or 4 drops carrier oil if your diffuser can
    handle a carrier oil without clogging

MEMORY IMPROVEMENT BLEND

One:

1 oz. carrier oil

2 drops peppermint essential oil

3 drops lemon essential oil

1 drop melissa essential oil

Use as a massage oil blend

Two:

1 oz. carrier oil

2 drops basil essential oil

1 drop rosemary essential oil

2 drops cedarwood essential oil

1 drop sandalwood essential oil

1 drop palo santo essential oil

Use as a massage oil blend

For Diffuser:

2 drops basil essential oil

2 drops rosemary essential oil

1 drop melissa essential oil

1 drop lemon essential oil

3 drops carrier oil if your diffuser can
    handle a carrier oil without clogging

Panic Blend
One:

1 oz. carrier oil

1 drop rose essential oil

4 drops lavender essential oil

1 drop frankincense essential oil

Use as a massage oil blend

Two:

1 oz. carrier oil

2 drops helichrysum essential oil

3 drops frankincense essential oil

1 drop lavender essential oil

Use as a massage oil blend

For Diffuser:

Use above blend proportions

Add 3 drops carrier oil if your diffuser can
    handle a carrier oil without clogging

Peace Blend

1 oz. carrier oil

7 drops Roman chamomile essential oil

5 drops lavender essential oil

1 drop palo santo essential oil

Use as a massage oil blend

For Diffuser:

2 drops Roman chamomile essential oil

1 drop lavender essential oil

1 drop geranium essential oil

4 drops carrier oil if your diffuser can handle a carrier oil without clogging

Strength Blend

One:

1 oz. carrier oil

3 drops myrrh essential oil

2 drops cedarwood essential oil

2 drops melissa essential oil

1 drop lemon essential oil

Use as a massage oil blend

Two:

1 oz. carrier oil

4 drops melissa essential oil

2 drops palo santo essential oil

1 drop myrrh essential oil

Use as a massage oil blend

For Diffuser:

2 drops cedarwood essential oil

2 drops palo santo essential oil

2 drops lemon essential oil

4 drops carrier oil if your diffuser can
    handle a carrier oil without clogging

SELF-CONFIDENCE BLEND
One:
1 oz. carrier oil

2 drops melissa essential oil

2 drops orange essential oil

1 drop pink grapefruit essential oil

1 drop sandalwood essential oil

2 drops bergamot essential oil

Use as a massage oil blend

Two:
1 oz. carrier oil

3 drops clary sage essential oil

1 drop lemon essential oil

2 drops vetiver essential oil

1 drop frankincense essential oil

1 drop rosemary essential oil

1 drop rose essential oil

Use as a massage oil blend

For Diffuser:
1 drop lemon essential oil

2 drops lemongrass essential oil

2 drops rosemary essential oil

3 drops carrier oil if your diffuser can
    handle a carrier oil without clogging

STRESS-REDUCTION BLEND

One:

1 oz. carrier oil

3 drops bergamot essential oil

1 drop geranium essential oil

1 drop frankincense essential oil

1 drop ylang-ylang essential oil

1 drop ravensara essential oil

Use as a massage oil blend

Two:

1 oz. carrier oil

3 drops pink grapefruit essential oil

1 drop rose essential oil

1 drop ylang-ylang essential oil

Use as a massage oil blend

For Diffuser:

3 drops pink grapefruit essential oil

1 drop lavender essential oil

1 drop ravensara essential oil

1 drop ylang-ylang essential oil

3 drops carrier oil if your diffuser can
   handle a carrier oil without clogging

WORKAHOLIC BLEND

One:

1 oz. carrier oil

2 drops geranium essential oil

2 drops lavender essential oil

1 drop basil essential oil

1 drop neroli essential oil

1 drop sandalwood essential oil

Use as a massage oil blend

Two:

1 oz. carrier oil

2 drops marjoram essential oil

1 drop basil essential oil

1 drop lavender essential oil

1 drop geranium essential oil

1 drop pink grapefruit essential oil

Use as a massage oil blend

For Diffuser:

2 drops geranium essential oil

2 drops lavender essential oil

1 drop basil essential oil

1 drop ylang-ylang essential oil

3 drops carrier oil if your diffuser can
    handle a carrier oil without clogging

As you work with the essential oils you will gain more expertise and creativity every day. Some blends will not resonate with you. Others will be spot on. Nobody knows you like you do. It really helps if you make notes as you go along so you'll remember the scents you like and those you don't.

The blends will speak to you and you can modify them as you and your nose decide. It can take time for essential oils to grow on you. Remember when you were a kid and you probably didn't like some vegetables? As you matured, your taste buds changed and maybe you even came to like them … a lot.

Give your brain a chance to integrate the smells and aromas with the results you feel. You may actually evolve into some of the scents as your body responds and as the natural essences of the essential oils grow on you. I wasn't fond of the heavier, muskier scents when I began, but now I appreciate them more each time I use them in a blend.

TWELVE

Sacred Uses of Essential Oils Throughout History

As far back as five thousand years ago, essential oils were used in sacred acts of purifying, consecrating, anointing, honoring, warding off evil spirits, summoning divine powers, conjuring spells, and bringing healing and comfort to the sick and injured.

Anointing

To be anointed means to have aromatic oil poured over your head (or entire body) or being doused or having a perfumed agent or product applied to your head, neck, or body. Anointing, used as a form of healing and as early medicine, was thought to drive out dangerous spirits and demons which were attributed to be the causes of all disease.

To anoint (from the Latin *inunctus*—"to smear with oil") means to make a person sacred, to set them apart and dedicate them to serve a higher spiritual purpose. In fact, the Bible refers to the use of anointing oils more than 150 times, and the Hebrew word *messiah* and the Greek word *christos* literally mean "anointed one."[321]

In present day usage, anointing is typically used for ceremonial blessings, but the tradition is ancient, honored, and filled with significance.

Anointing, particularly the anointing of the sick and the anointing of the dying, are major components of last rites in the Catholic church, called extreme unction.

---

321   Dennis William Hauck, "History of Essential Oils," crucible.org/oils_history.htm.

Applications of oils and fats are also historically used in traditional medicines. Olive oil was frequently used on wounds and applied to the sick. Centuries of demons have been fought off using ritualized oils.

They are still used in traditional Indian medicine to remove illness, bad luck, and demonic possession. Anointing is also believed to act as a sacred seal and goodness.

Throughout history the practice of anointing the dead was done to protect the corpse against evil spirits and for sanitation.

If you were a guest in ancient Egypt you would be greeted and anointed with a special oil as you entered a private home. Some Arab families still observe this practice today. Persian Zoroastrians honor their visitors with rose extract while holding a mirror in front of their guest's face to let them know they are welcome. The words *rooj kori aka* ("have a nice day") are spoken aloud, during a custom that is nearly three thousand years old.[322]

Also in ancient Egypt, anointing was depicted as a private moment between husband and wife. In ancient Egypt when the wife anointed her spouse it was a sign of affection and an intimate moment. There are drawings on the throne of Tutankhamen depicting such anointing rituals.

Vedic rituals involved the anointing of government officials, worshippers, and idols now known as *abhisheka*. The anointing practice was adopted by Indian Buddhists. They use water, yoghurt, milk, or butter from blessed cows rather than oil. Devotees are consecrated and blessed at every stage of life. Rituals are performed for birth, education, initiations, marriage, and death. New buildings, houses, and ritual instruments are anointed, and some idols are even anointed daily.

The Roman Catholic and Anglican churches bless three types of holy oils for anointing: Oil of the Catechumens (abbreviated OS, from the Latin *oleum sanctum*), Oil of the Infirm (OI), and Sacred Chrism (SC).

The Oil of Catechumens is used to anoint the catechumens (adults preparing for reception into the church) just before their receipt of the sacrament of baptism.[323] The Oil of the Inform is used to anoint the sick and turn the healing over to the Lord for restoration of health. The Sacred Chrism is used in the sacraments of baptism, confirmation, and holy orders.

---

322 "Anointment," www.revolvy.com/main/index.php?s=Anointment&item_type=topic.

323 "Holy Oils," www.fisheaters.com/holyoils.html.

Crosses are traditionally not considered holy until they have been anointed and prayed over in the Armenian church. The act of anointing introduces the Holy Spirit into them.

Pentecostal churches, who are centered in the Holy Spirit, anoint and consecrate their pastors and elders. The sick are also anointed when healed.

Founder Joseph Smith instituted anointing for the rites of sanctification and consecration practiced in the temples of the Latter-day Saints. Presently, any member of the Melchizedek priesthood may anoint the head of an individual with olive oil if they are ill. Only olive oil must be used and it must be consecrated by a Melchizedek priest.

Anointing has been an important ritual at European coronations, both historically and in legend. French legend has it that a vial of oil—the Holy Ampulla—descended from heaven to anoint Clovis I as king of the Franks following his conversion to Christianity in 493 CE.[324]

In Eastern Orthodoxy, the anointing of a new king is considered a sacred mystery. The act is believed to empower him to perform his divinely appointed duties, using the grace of the Holy Spirit to defend the faith. In Russian tradition ceremonial anointing took place during the coronation of the tsar toward the end of the service, just before his receipt of communion.

In the present day, royal unction is less common, but is still practiced by the rulers of Britain and of Tonga.

Here are some other examples of plants and oils used in rituals and for anointing:

Cedarwood (*Cedrus atlantica*) used in ritual purification after touching anything unclean.

Chamomile (*Anthemis nobilis*) was considered a sacred herb by the Egyptians, Moors, and Saxons.

Clary sage (*Salvia sclarea*) or "sacred herb," *herba sacra*, regarded as such by the Romans because of its euphoric properties.

---

324   Ralph E. Giesey, ed. Sean Wilentz, "Models of Rulership in French Royal Ceremonial" in *Rites of Power: Symbolism, Ritual, and Politics Since the Middle Ages* (Philadelphia: University of Philadelphia Press, 1985), 43.

Fennel (*Foeniculum vulgare*) was thought to ward off evil spirits and spells cast by witches. Sprigs of fennel were hung over doorways to fend off evil.

Galbanum (*Ferula galbaniflua*) was considered spiritually uplifting.

Hyssop (*Hyssopus officinalis var.*) was used to protect against plague and to drive away evil spirits.

Juniper (*Juniperus communis L.*) was used in the Middle Ages to ward off witches.

Marjoram (*Origanum majorana*) was considered a funeral herb to bring spiritual peace to the departed.

Melissa (Lemon Balm) (*Melissa officinalis*) was considered the "elixir of life" and used to reduce nervousness and ailments dealing with the heart, anxiety, melancholy, and to strengthen and revive the vital inner spirit.

Mugwort (*Artemisia herba-alba*) was associated with superstition and witchcraft and was used as a protective charm against evil and danger in the Middle Ages.

Myrrh (*Commiphora myrrha*) is one of the oldest spiritual oils regarded as elevating humans to the spirit of the gods.

Myrtle (*Myrtus communis*) was considered a sign of immortality and used in religious ceremonies.

Palo santo (*Bursera graveolens*) was known to peoples of Latin America as a spiritual oil used to purify and cleanse the air of negative energies.

Sage (*Salvia officinalis*) was used by native peoples to help cleanse the ethers of negativity.

Sandalwood (*Santalum*) is considered one of the oldest oils known for its spiritual qualities and assistance with prayer and meditation.

Spikenard (*Nardostachys grandiflora*) was considered one of the sacred chrisms for anointing monarchs and high initiates into the mystery schools.[325]

---

325 *Chrism* is an ancient word for consecrated oil used to anoint in baptism and other special sacraments.

Black spruce (*Picea mariana*) used by the Lakota Indians to strengthen their ability to communicate with the Great Spirit. They believed spruce possessed the frequency of prosperity.

Thyme (*Thymus vulgaris*) was associated with courage. The Roman soldiers bathed in thyme before going into battle, and in the Middle Ages sprigs of thyme were woven into the scarves of knights departing for the Crusades—again, to boost courage.

Yarrow (*Achillea millefolium*) in the Middle Ages was traditionally cut with a black-handled knife in the moonlight, over which mystic words were repeated. It was then placed under the pillow so that young girls would dream of their true loves.[326]

You may not have thought to use essential oils for sacred purposes, but consider this: initiations, ceremonies, rituals, and rites of passage have been marked with essential oil usage for centuries. You can incorporate them into your life and celebrate the chapters of your growth and progress by using any essential oil that seems appropriate for you or the event.

If you would like to enrich your life through the practice of anointing, here is a list of suggested milestones and markers that you may want to ritualize by using diluted essential oils.

You can integrate essential oils into your own rituals to celebrate and commemorate:

Academic: First day, graduations, commencements, honors, good grades

Birthdays: Quinceañera, sweet sixteen, turning twenty-one, milestone ages

Firsts: House, school, new bike, new job, promotion

Loss: Honoring the transition of a loved one, pet, or any loss of any kind

Lunar events: Monthly phases of the moon, lunar eclipses

---

326   Linda Lee Smith, "Essential Oils—19 'Magical' Plants For Warding Off Evil," ezinearticles .com/?Essential-Oils—19–Magical-Plants-For-Warding-Off-Evil&id=1319468.

New baby: Baptism, christening, brit milah (bris), baby naming, (make sure you follow the guidelines about pregnancy and essential oils in the chapter on Cautions)

Romance: Engagement, marriage, anniversary

Solar events: Summer and winter solstices, autumnal and spring equinox

Other: Successful surgery, transplant, winnings

Rituals

Many religious practices use sacred oils in their scripted rituals. This list here is not meant to usurp any beliefs or practices, only to add even more depth to life as a celebration and an experience of joy.

Create a Ritual

1. Choose a meaningful occasion you wish to make special.

2. Select an appropriate location for the anointing.

3. Make sure you have a willing anointee.

4. Write an opening statement of purpose and intention: Why you are selecting this time or event as special?

5. Write a positive and affirming short statement about the reasons why this day, person, achievement, event is important and worth commemorating.

6. Use an essential oil or oils you feel have the qualities that represent this person or event, or the qualities you wish to impart. (You can use the list in this chapter or select from the lists and descriptions of essential oils from previous chapters.) Be sure you dilute all essential oils before using.

7. End with a blessing, a prayer, a poem, or any closing you feel is appropriate to this ritual.

Sample Ritual Scripts

Anointing is, in essence, an honoring and celebration of life. It can be used to honor milestones or passages or to highlight and deepen the significance of joyful occasions. I offer here a few sample anointing ceremonies, trusting that they might inspire you to celebrate and create some of your own.

BIRTHDAYS

Birthdays are a wonderful opportunity to honor someone with an anointing ceremony, especially those birthdays that mark major milestones in a person's life: Quinceañera, twenty-first birthday, the decades (thirty, forty, fifty, etc.). In this example, the person being celebrated turns twenty-one.

Opening statement:
"We are here today to celebrate (Name) and to acknowledge the significance of this wonderful day, in which (Name) becomes twenty-one. This birthday is particularly important because twenty-one is the age at which our society says a person has become an adult. Along with the rights, responsibilities, and privileges that the government bestows upon an adult, there is also the recognition, by family, friends, and the world at large that (Name) is responsible now for his/her own words and actions and is officially authorized to fully participate in life trusting in the wisdom and knowledge that he/she has learned from those who have been his/her teachers, mentors, and guides."

Say while anointing:
"(Name), as we honor you today I anoint you with a blend of rosemary for longevity, thyme for courage, myrrh so that your spirit may always be lifted to the highest level, and rose so your days may always be filled with love, peace, and beauty."

Closing statement:
"(Name), we have watched you learn and grow for twenty-one years and during that time we have celebrated many of the special events and adventures that have brought you to this moment. We have been honored, entertained,

and delighted by your progress these first twenty-one years and it has been a joy to watch the child you have been become the man/woman that you are today. And today we honor, acknowledge, and celebrate the adult that you have become. In the years to come may your wisdom be a guiding light for others; may your love make our world a kinder place; and may we be blessed by your presence for many decades to come." (You may wish to add a prayer to the ending if that is appropriate for your gathering.)

Engagement or Marriage

Love and romance create many moments that are ideal for anointing. You might consider taking a few moments at the beginning of a bridal shower to anoint the bride-to-be with special blessings from her friends and family. Or perhaps you might create a special moment with both the bride- and groom-to-be and do a private anointing to bless their future together. With their permission and that of the officiant, of course, an anointing during the wedding ceremony itself could be a magical and meaningful moment, or (again, with their permission) an essential oil blessing pre-arranged in a private setting just after the ceremony and before they are surrounded by well-wishers and the photographer.

This sample ceremony might take place with close friends immediately after the engagement is announced, at the beginning of a wedding shower for the couple in which both bride and groom are present, or any time or place that feels right and appropriate to the engaged couple.

One person can do the anointing ceremony or a group of people (perhaps the bridal party or close family members) can each anoint the couple with a drop of a specially selected essential oil. The couple may sit or stand together in the center of a circle formed by their loved ones.

Opening statement:
The abundant blessings of love have already fallen upon (names of couple) and your lives will never be quite the same. You have pledged your hearts to one another and there is no magic more powerful than that. But today we who love you would like to take a few moments and add our individual wishes and blessings to your already overflowing cup of love.

We ask you stand (or sit) together and hold one another's hand—and open your free hand and your hearts to receive our gifts.

Each anointing person now comes to the couple with a vial of specially selected essential oil and places a drop of the oil on each of their hands. As they place the oil on the couple's hands a blessing is said.

Say while anointing:
(Examples of possible blessings, feel free to choose any oils and blessings that are appropriate for the couple/people involved.)

I anoint you with rosemary, that you may live long together.

I anoint you with rose, that you may always live in love and peace and that beauty may always surround you.

I anoint you with tea tree, that you may always live in harmony.

I anoint you with clove bud, that you may always have the energy and desire to make love. May your life together always be spicy.

I anoint you with bergamot essential oil, may your life be abundant in all ways.

Closing statement:
May these many blessings stay in your hearts and your lives for many decades to come and may they remain vivid in your memory so that you know our love is with you always. We would also like to give you this gift of a diffuser of essential oils and a vial of (name of specific essential oil(s) i.e., geranium or a combination of oils) that your house may always be filled with protection, happiness, and love.

A prayer for the couple may conclude the anointing if that is appropriate.

New Baby

Note: Be sure you follow the cautions in chapter five and use age-appropriate dilutions for use with children and infants.

The birth of a baby is a joyous time celebrated with showers both before and after the actual event. While the baby is too young and sensitive to have oils applied, this could be a wonderful time to anoint the mother and/or father of the child and bless their lives with the gifts that essential oils bring.

Opening statement:

In the whirlwind of activity that surrounds the birth of a baby it is easy to forget to take the time to nurture and support the baby's parents. Today we take a moment and, like fairy godmothers with gifts to bestow, honor this new father and mother and anoint them with oils that will give them the attributes that every new parent needs.

(Name/s), we take a few moments today to honor and support you. You have many wonderful and exciting times—and sleepless nights—ahead of you as this child grows into the wonderful person we know he/she will become. And we can know that he/she will be wonderful because you will share your wisdom, love, knowledge, and heart and soul with him/her as he/she grows through the stages of his/her life.

Each anointing person now comes to the couple with a vial of specially selected essential oil and places a drop of the oil on each of their hands. As they place the oil on the couple's hands a blessing is said.

Say while anointing:

(Examples of possible blessings; feel free to choose any oils and blessings that are appropriate for the family involved.)

I anoint you with basil, that your beautiful family may always find peace and happiness.

I anoint you with Roman chamomile, so you will sleep well when you can and dream the sweetest dreams.

I anoint you with rosemary, so that you will attract the prosperity to fund your dreams for this child.

I anoint you with orange, so that you may always be vigilant in caring for this child.

I anoint you with lemon, that you are blessed with abundant energy and great wit as this child grows and challenges you.

I anoint you with neroli, that you may know that your family is blessed and protected.

Closing statement:
May these many blessings remain in your memory as this child grows and teaches you about things you may never have known you didn't know. May you find wisdom, peace, and comfort in them and may they continue to bless your lives through all of the wonderful experiences ahead of you. Remember the gifts that have been bestowed upon you today and know that they go with you throughout your lives.

We would like to present you with these bottles of essential oils in the hope that you will use them in the future to find extra strength, lightness, and wisdom when they are needed; and to find restful sleep in the days and nights to come.

A prayer for the couple may conclude the anointing if that is appropriate.

HOUSEWARMING

Moving into a new home is always a special occasion and with friends and love ones gathered around, a great opportunity to bless both the house and its new occupants. It is also a good time to "clean house" of any past energies that no longer belong there and to make room for the new family and its happy future.

Opening statement:
What a happy day this is! (Names of new home owners) are moving into their new home and we are here to celebrate and bless this wonderful new beginning.

This is an exciting time, the start of a new adventure, the foundation of the next chapter in their lives together. Their lives will be lived out under this roof. Decisions will be made at this table that effect their future. A family will learn and grow within these walls and we all wish our friends years of peace, safety, and happiness here. Many celebrations will be held in this house, many milestones will be marked; we expect that there will be many opportunities to celebrate joy here. But before we go on with today's celebration, we take a few minutes to acknowledge and bless the role this house will play in our friends' lives in the coming years.

Take a small vial of diluted essential oil(s) and walk from room to room placing a small drop of oil in a corner of each room in the house while saying a word or two of blessing appropriate for each room. For example, while anointing in:

The kitchen:
May the food prepared in this room always nourish those who eat here. May it build strong bodies and inspire wise and peaceful minds and may there always be plenty in this house. This essential oil blend contains melissa, lemon balm, the 'elixir of life' so that the food served in this room will build strength and revive the energies of those who live here.

The bedroom:
"May love abide here. May the day end gently here. May the nights be peaceful and may sleep come easily. And may every morning be welcomed with a smile of gratitude for another day of love and joy and prosperity for this family. This essential oil blend contains tea tree essential oil for harmony; rose for love, peace, and beauty; and sandalwood essential oil, which not only enhances your times of prayer and meditation but as an aphrodisiac, makes love even more exciting in this space."

The family room:
"Life happens here. This family room is dedicated to the growth of this family in every area of their lives. The essential oils we place here are vetiver essential oil for protection, sage to cleanse, and myrrh to lift and enlighten their journey. May they grow strong and wise, both individually and together, in this space. May they learn respect and appreciation for one another in this place. May they come to greater understanding of the unique gifts of each of the members of this family and may they grow in love within these walls and may that love reach beyond these walls to touch and bless the lives of others."

When you have processed through the entire house saying a special sentence of blessing in each room return to the room in which you started.

To conclude:
This is a new beginning. With the essential oils of clary sage we cleanse the ethers of any past negativity, with bergamot and rose essential oils we infuse this space with joy, love, peace and beauty. Today we cleanse this house of any remnants of the past that it may be free to provide only blessings for this family.

Additional option:
Put essential oils in a diffuser and place it in the room in which you conclude, saying:

We leave a diffuser with essential oils in this room so that the air in this house will remain alive with these blessings and intentions. (Be sure to follow the cautions in chapter five for diffusing around children and pets.)

Conclude by saying:
"With these sacred essential oils we put into motion energies that vitalize and renew each day. May times of joy be multiplied many times over. May opportunities abound within these walls and may the occasional moments of sadness, sorrow, or concern be washed away by the tears of love and the soothing sound of laughter." (You may also wish to add a prayer to the ending if that is appropriate for your gathering.)

Create rituals and anointing practices to enrich and enhance your life and to bring meaning to the passages of your life and the lives of your cherished friends and family. You may want to make a special notebook or scrapbook containing the rituals for your family that can be passed down generationally.

THIRTEEN

Alternative Methods for Using Essential Oils for Healing

Everything is possible. All goals can be achieved. All wounds can be healed and all negativity can be exchanged for something more positive and life-affirming. The art of healing is deep within the body and resides there genetically and spiritually. It is never impossible to heal anything and everything in your mind, body, and spirit. When you set your mind and intention to healing, you create an energy that sets the therapy in motion immediately and you awaken the healer within.

Once you make up your mind to heal, pathways open up and appear in your life like summer fruit hanging on a branch primed for picking. It is no longer a question of *if* you are going to heal, but a question of *how* you are going to heal. What method will you use, or what approach will you take given all the alternatives you have to choose from? Is there one system that will offer you the best inspiration and the structure for your healing process? Like fingerprints, people are different. Tastes are varied and one size does not fit all. Do you prefer to stick to the more traditional methods or are you one who likes to experiment with new approaches? There are many paths we can take.

I'd like to share with you a few different ways you can use the essential oils. The first method comes from ancient teachings and uses the energy fields of the body. Essential oils are paired with each of the seven chakras and healing can occur as you use the guidelines to locate your issues, work with the essential oils associated with a chakra, and move up through the circles of spiraling energy.

Chakra Healing

Understanding how the seven chakras work allows you to discover the relationship between your consciousness and your body and subsequently helps you to balance what is making you feel out of sorts or what is causing you pain and distress. The seven chakras are an effective way to access the roadmap of your body because they show you, in clear terms, what you are thinking, feeling, and experiencing, and even tell you *why*. The seven chakras healing system gives you a better understanding of yourself and those around you. Essential oils can help you balance them to attain relief or stimulation as you need it for each area.

The word *chakra* is Sanskrit for "vortex," "spinning wheel," or "circle." According to Vedic beliefs, chakras are circles of energy that balance, store, and distribute the energies of life all through our physical body via the subtle body, the nonphysical body otherwise known as our soul or spirit overlaying the physical body.

The practice of healing by attending to the chakras originated in India as an Ayurvedic medicine (*ayur* meaning life and *veda* meaning knowledge) practice, dating back to 2500 BCE. The word "ayurveda" can also be interpreted as knowledge for leading a balanced and healthy life. You may discover that this method is an effective way to monitor what is really going on with you on the physical and spiritual planes.

Picture the seven chakras as circles of energy flowing throughout your body. These energetic circles assist in the running of your body, mind, and soul. If one chakra or another is not performing correctly, you can experience negative effects in your physical, mental, or spiritual health.

Chakras are not actually physical; they are aspects of consciousness, but the body responds to the negative or positive energy of the chakra and the physical manifestations of chakra energy are real and measurable. The chakras are not as dense as the physical body; they interact with the physical body through two major passageways: the endocrine system and the nervous system.[327] Each chakra can be associated with a particular part of the body and certain physical functions within the body. Working in tandem, the chakras represent not only individual parts of your material body, but also particular parts of your consciousness.

---

327   Timothy Pope, "Chakras and the Endocrine System," http://www.healingfromtheheart
       .co.uk/69701.html.

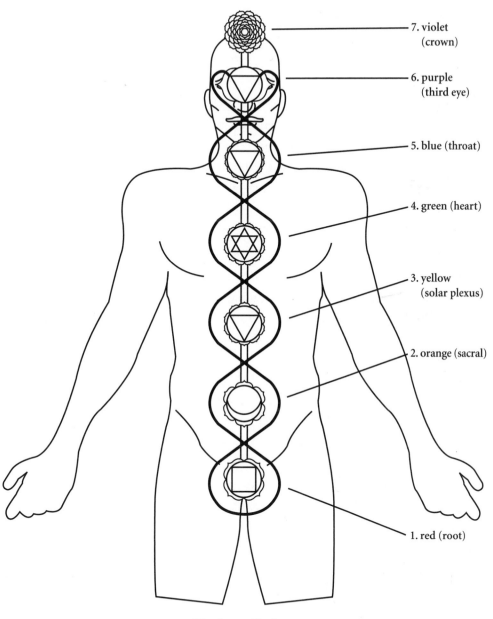

7. violet
(crown)

6. purple
(third eye)

5. blue (throat)

4. green (heart)

3. yellow
(solar plexus)

2. orange (sacral)

1. red (root)

The Seven Chakras

These seven chakras, or energy wheels, start at the base of the spine and move upward to the seventh area located at the crown of the head. They coincide with the positions along the spinal cord of the major nerve groups in our physical body. Each chakra not only represents a particular part of the body, a natural element, and a separate color and qualities attributed to it, but also represents a musical tone or note. The universe is frequently referred to as the "uni-verse," that is, one song made up of many sounds.[328] The sounds embodied by the seven chakras comprise a musical harmony for the triad of mind, body, and spirit.

Following is a breakdown of what the seven key chakras represent and how they can affect your emotional and spiritual life when assisted by essential oils.

The First Chakra: The Root Chakra (Muladhara)

Color: Red

Location: The base of the spine, *muladhara,* is associated with stability, ambition, financial independence, and grounding and centering. It is the hub of our immune system and represents our survival (food, shelter, protection) and early family ties. It is the chakra from which action and vitality originate.

Balanced: We feel alive, optimistic, happy, strong, grounded, vital, motivated, and powerful.

Imbalanced: We may experience depression, confusion, alienation, self-centeredness, jealousy, aggression, or rage. Without a balance of this chakra the other six chakras will not be able to function correctly.

Body: Legs, bones, adrenal glands, colon, spinal column.

Element: Earth

Musical note: C

Suggested essential oils: Cedarwood, frankincense, myrrh, melissa, neroli, palo santo, patchouli, sandalwood, spikenard, vetiver.

---

328 Erin Johnson, "The Universe as One Mind," scienceblogs.com/revminds/2009/09/02/the-universe-as-one-song/.

The Second Chakra: The Sacral Chakra (Svadhisthana)

Color: Orange

Location: Lower abdomen, *svadhisthana,* is found just below the navel. It is the source of creativity and inspiration. It is the foundation of our emotions.

Balanced: We experience abundance, creativity, optimism, healthy sexuality, and overall well-being.

Imbalanced: We may feel irritable, shy, needy, withdrawn, hyper-sensitive, fearful of intimacy, or have sexual-related issues of impotence, frigidity, or infidelity.

Body: Lower abdomen, spleen, liver, bladder, kidneys, reproductive organs.

Element: Water

Musical note: D

Suggested essential oils: Ginger, cedarwood, sandalwood, ylang-ylang, clary sage, neroli, orange, patchouli, rose, bergamot, vetiver.

The Third Chakra: The Solar Plexus (Manipura)

Color: Yellow

Location: Centered in the upper abdomen.

Balanced: We feel solid in our self, tolerant of others, patient, positive, understanding, peaceful, intuitive, flexible, and clear in decision-making.

Imbalanced: We may feel under-confident, lacking in good judgment, abandoned, nervous, stressed, addicted, egocentric, conflicted, angry.

Body: Liver, spleen, gallbladder.

Element: Fire

Musical Note: E

Suggested essential oils: Cedarwood, cinnamon, clove bud, ginger, geranium, pink grapefruit, lemongrass, peppermint, rosemary, sandalwood, vetiver, ylang-ylang.

The Fourth Chakra: The Heart Chakra (Anahata)

Color: Green

Location: Heart area.

Balanced: We feel open, wise, forgiving, compassionate, prosperous, peaceful, humanitarian, and capable of unconditional love.

Imbalanced: We feel unstable, martyred, suspicious, repressed, unloved, lonely, jealous, and stingy.

Body: Heart, lungs, thymus, circulation, immune systems.

Element: Air

Musical note: F

Suggested essential oils: Bergamot, geranium, jasmine, lavender, lemon, melissa, neroli, orange, rose, sandalwood, ylang-ylang.

The Fifth Chakra: The Throat Chakra (Vishuddha)

Color: Blue

Location: Base of the neck, in the throat.

Balanced: We feel patient and honest, have open communication and emotional expressiveness, listen well, and positively receive constructive criticism.

Imbalanced: We feel inflexible, nervous, self-righteous, introverted, faithless, deceitful, dishonest, possibly addicted, and unable to communicate effectively.

Body: Thyroid, mouth, teeth, throat.

Elements: Ether and earth

Musical note: G

Suggested essential oils: Cedarwood, basil, bergamot, black pepper, clary sage, clove bud, helichrysum, lavender, peppermint, rose, roman chamomile, orange.

The Sixth Chakra: The Third Eye Chakra (**Ajna**)

Color: Indigo

Location: Forehead, between the eyebrows.

Balanced: We feel guided by a higher power, connected to our spiritual nature, trusting, trustworthy, clairvoyant, purpose-driven, intuitive.

Imbalanced: We feel confused, clingy, unassertive, judgmental, forgetful, unmotivated, egocentric, materialistic.

Body: Pituitary

Element: Water

Musical note: A

Suggested essential oils: Bergamot, benzoin, clary sage, frankincense, helichrysum, lemon, lemongrass, marjoram, neroli, patchouli, rosemary, sandalwood, vetiver.

The Seventh Chakra: The Crown Chakra (**Sahasrara**)

Color: White or violet

Location: Top of the head/crown.

Balanced: We feel unity with the universe, open-minded, spiritually centered, idealistic, trusting in a greater good, purpose-driven, wise, insightful, selfless.

Imbalanced: We feel devoid of spirit, fearful, alone, unloved, lacking purpose, forsaken, atheistic.

Body: Cerebral cortex, cerebrum, nervous system, pineal and pituitary glands.

Element: Thought

Musical note: B

Suggested essential oils: Cedarwood, frankincense, helichrysum, lavender, melissa, myrrh, neroli, palo santo, rose, sandalwood, spikenard, vetiver.

Self-Diagnosis

When you feel tension or negativity in your body or mind, you register it in one of the seven chakras associated with that part of your consciousness experiencing the stress. You'll probably even sense the discomfort in the parts of your physical body associated with a specific chakra. When you experience the emotion of joy or success, you'll also register it in one of the seven chakras. And you'll experience the freedom and lightness of the more positive emotions, too.

It is a highly beneficial practice to regularly check in with the seven chakras for evidence as to what is going on inside of you. If you catch an imbalance early, you can stabilize it before it causes you any real damage. You can also support superior chakra function by cultivating positive emotions, thoughts, qualities, and feelings that boost and enhance the chakras.

There are many ways you can use your seven chakras and several approaches you can take to keep them balanced and working together. You can use a checklist or make an appointment with an Ayurvedic doctor or practitioner. Or, you can meditate and ask yourself a few questions:

- How am I feeling right now?
- What are my physical feelings?
- My emotions?
- Am I happy?
- Am I at peace?
- Does my life work?
- Am I achieving what I want in my life?
- Am I surrounded by loving and supportive people?
- What do I need to change to have what I want?
- Are there any feelings I need to adjust?
- What is my spiritual life like?
- If I could change one thing right now, it would be_____.

Your answers will usually line up with one (or two) of the chakras and you can begin to heal using the essential oils recommended for that chakra. Strive for balance.

Five Element Healing

The next alternative method you may want to explore is taken from Chinese Medicine. It uses the Five Elements for achieving balance based in the natural cycles of creation and destruction.

The Chinese view is of the human body, personality, the environment, and nature through a core explanation of life called the Five Element system. Everything alive functions according to this system. The elements are: Wood, Fire, Earth, Metal, and Water.

A simple chart explains the natural cycles the body and the emotions sequence throughout the various phases and seasons in a twelve-month rotation.

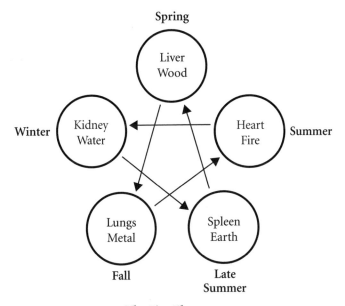

The Five Elements

- Each season "rules" organs, emotions, and body parts.
- Each season has certain attributes, qualities, and overriding natural energies.

- Each season has certain colors, textures, and shapes associated with it.

- Each season has organ systems and meridians of energy associated with it.

- Each season has certain clues and body cues to let you know when it's out of balance.

When you utilize the Five Elements to test your inner and outer balance, you will find ways to bring about the cycle of natural support using the essential oils. The elements, when balanced, will keep you healthy and humming along. The Chinese believe that when you have achieved a balance between the Five Elements in your body and your environment you will experience harmony.

Seasons

SUMMER

Element: Fire

Energy: Yang

Color: Red

Body part(s)/meridians: Small Intestine, Heart, Pericardium

Clues of Imbalance:

Overly excitable

Inability to relax

ADD

Hyperactivity

Manic episodes

Chronic tension

Manifestation:

High blood pressure

Shoulder and neck pain

Flushed complexion

Light headedness

Heart palpitations

Poor circulation

Frozen shoulder
Chest pain
Dark circles under eyes
Hardening of the arteries
Hearing difficulties
Herpes
High or low blood sugar
Cold sores
Confusion
Constipation
Diarrhea
Dry hair and skin
Indigestion
Mouth ulcers
Pimples
Poor circulation
Fatigue
Depression
Anxiety
Aversion to heat
Insomnia

Essential Oils:
Rose
Neroli
Cinnamon
Lavender
Lemon
Lemongrass
Marjoram
Ylang-ylang
Black pepper

Ginger
Cedarwood
Sandalwood

When Fire is balanced the qualities of dynamism, strength, and persistence are present. The Fire element provides, warmth, enthusiasm, and creativity. It also brings heat and warmth and is responsible for the passionate resonance you feel when you are following your life's calling. Fire is the joy and laughter associated with playfulness and accomplishment.

LATE SUMMER
Element: Earth
Energy: Yin/yang balance
Color: Yellow
Body part(s)/meridians: Spleen, pancreas, stomach

Clues of Imbalance:
Erratic energy levels
Sweet tooth
Arthritis
Heartburn
Indigestion
Shoulder and neck tension
Stomach ulcer
Sinusitis
Eczema
Rashes
Food allergies
Diabetes
Poor lymph circulation
Frequent urination
Low blood sugar
Insomnia

Bed wetting

Sciatica

Constipation

Uterine

Prostate

Hemorrhoids

Obesity

Manifestation:

Mood swings

Jealousy

Hyper-sensitivity

Anxiety

Essential Oils:

Geranium

Rose

Rosemary

Patchouli

Myrrh

Vetiver

Cedarwood

Sandalwood

Ginger

Marjoram

Lavender

Ylang-ylang

When Earth is in balance both yin and yang, the feminine and masculine, work together. The energy is inward, centering, stabilizing, and conserving. The turning of the seasons represents Earth and fosters the qualities of practicality, patience, hard work, thoughtfulness, and stability. The energy of Earth energy is that of a mother and likes to bring everything together with a sense of order to establish harmony.

Fall

Element: Metal

Energy: Yin

Color: White

Body part(s)/meridians: Lungs, large intestine

Clues of Imbalance:

Sinuses/mucus/phlegm

Cardio-vascular problems

Respiratory issues

Allergies

Heart disease

Asthma

Lung cancer

Breast cancer

Intestinal/digestive issues

Thoracic spine issues

Pneumonia

Hypertension

Stroke

Pale complexion

Angina

Arthritis

Shoulder girdle pain and discomfort

Rotator cuff injuries

Tendonitis

Carpal tunnel

Arm and hand pain

Manifestation:

Sadness

Depression

Melancholy

Apathy

Weariness

Insensitivity

Anxiety

Emotionally distant

Unforgiving

Essential Oils:

Cinnamon

Clove bud

Ginger

Tea Tree

Thyme

Coriander

Eucalyptus

Marjoram

Lemongrass

Ravensara

Myrrh

Frankincense

Spikenard

Ylang-ylang

Yarrow

When the Metal element is balanced, the breath of life is active present. When you are connected to primal breath you appreciate your own personal power and self-worth. You have respect for yourself and for others and you participate in exchange that is beneficial to all for a vibrant life. You possess structure, stability, appreciation, and flexibility.

WINTER

Element: Water

Energy: Yin

Color: Black/Dark Blue

Body part(s)/meridians: Kidneys, bladder, reproductive organs

Clues of Imbalance:

Leg pain

Lumbar tension

Low back pain

Chronic fatigue

Claustrophobic

Underarm and foot odor

Hammer and pigeon toes

Low or high blood sugar

Bed wetting

Always cold

Pale urine

Kidney and bladder infection

Immune disorders

Skin conditions

Swelling and edema

Sweaty palms and feet

Low energy

Chronically stressed

Impatience

Dark circles under eyes

Salt craving

Sensitive to cold

Impotence

Frigidity

Irritable bowel

Painful urination

Cystitis

Urinary tract infection

Sciatica

Tight hamstrings

Prostate conditions
Addictions of all kinds

Manifestation:
Overwhelmed
Timid
Insecure
Fearful
Easily frightened

Essential oils:
Bergamot
Geranium
Neroli
Orange
Rose
Lavender
Clary sage
Ylang-ylang

When the Water element is in balance in the body resources are allocated well and used wisely. Life is a series of exchanges of time, contacts, resources, talents, ideas and money. Nothing is retained or squandered; all is kept in the flow and balance of natural, sustaining exchange. Water is the element of stillness; it requires rest. When water is balanced there is enough time to rejuvenate before taking action. The Water element provides time to innovate and create new ideas.

Spring
Element: Wood
Energy: Yang (beginning)
Color: Green
Body part(s)/meridians: Liver, gallbladder

Clues of Imbalance:

Abdominal bloating

Digestive upsets

Breast tenderness

Cellulite

Coated tongue

Constipation

Excessive bleeding

Gout

Red eyes

Irregular and painful menses

Fatigue

Flatulence

Gall Stones

Halitosis

Headaches

Hemorrhoids

Hepatitis

Leg edema

Nausea

Soft nails

Stiff neck and shoulders

Skin conditions

Varicose veins

Uterine fibroids

Tendency to overeat

Manifestation:

Anger

Domination

Frustration

Criticism

Essential Oils:
Basil
Sandalwood
Cedarwood
Geranium
Lemon
Lemongrass
Lavender
Rosemary
Spikenard
Palo santo

When the Wood element is balanced the leader within us takes charge and determines a solid course of action. Our life moves forward. Wood seeks to grow and expand. It announces the beginning of new life, springtime, sensuality, and growth.

Use this information to check in with the symptoms, assess your condition in terms of yin/yang, or balance of the element.

How to Use the Five Elements for Healing

Using this Chinese Medicine principle we are going to *tonify,* which means to impart tone to the body parts/meridians by using essential oils to soothe what is overactive or stimulate what is lacking.

1. First, make a list of your symptoms, ailments, or discomforts—those things you are experiencing and would like to alleviate.

2. Compare your symptoms against the list of manifestations for each of the seasons noted above. If you have five or more of the clues or manifestations, you are out of balance with the ruling element and season. You will proceed to create a better balance using essential oils.

3. Check your symptoms or manifestations with the list of emotions in chapter eleven.

4. Select the essential oils recommended for the emotion or condition that registers for you and make a massage blend, a diffuser blend, an inhaler or any other uses for essential oils suggested in chapter fourteen.

5. Use the essential oil remedy for five days, then recheck your symptoms and physical manifestation again and rate your improvement.

6. If there is room for more improvement, repeat the process and maybe add in another essential oil or two as your intuition guides you.

7. Use again for five days and recheck for improvement. If the condition persists, changes, worsens, or does not respond to these essential oil blends, you may need to seek medical help.

Astrological Healing

Another effective alternative approach to healing is to utilize your astrological sign as a guideline.

We are often amused by our horoscope and don't take it more seriously than a fortune cookie message read after dinner at our local Chinese restaurant.

However, we can discover a lot about ourselves through astrological sciences, our natal sign, the time of our birth, the placement of the sun, the moon, and our rising sign at the moment we entered life.

It is not recommended that you use this information as superstition, but rather a light source illuminating the landscape of your life. When you know what aspects you were given at birth, you possess a special knowledge to help you along your path.

Read about the astrological signs and the qualities and characteristics that accompany your birth date. You will discover that they have certain values, strengths, and weaknesses and there will be signs of balance and imbalance.

You are one of twelve possibilities. Everyone in the world is one sign or another.

If you were born March 21–April 19, you are an

ARIES

Planetary ruler: Mars

Element: Fire

Key phrase: "I am"

Beneficial traits: Active, demanding, determined, effective, courageous, ambitious, confident, enthusiastic, passionate, fiery, frank, exciting, energetic, curious, and competitive

Challenging traits: Arrogant, impatient, domineering, easily bored, argumentative, impulsive, prefers to lead rather than to be led

Body parts: Head, brain, and eyes; caution for headaches and stress-related problems

Essential oils: Black pepper, frankincense, lemon, and rosemary support Aries' nature; peppermint, rose, and marjoram are excellent for calming the fire element; Roman chamomile and lavender are useful in alleviating a strong head

If you were born April 20–May 20, you are a

TAURUS

Planetary ruler: Venus

Element: Earth

Key phrase: "I have"

Beneficial traits: Steady and strong, appreciative of beauty, patient, long-suffering, kind, gentle, reliable

Challenging traits: Jealous, greedy, possessive, materialistic, opinionated, stubborn

Body parts: Throat, cerebellum, thyroid; prone to sore throats, overindulgence, colds, stiff necks

Essential oils: Black pepper, rosemary, lemon for aching muscles; eucalyptus and Roman chamomile for sore throats; and patchouli and ylang-ylang for the sensual side

If you were born May 21–June 20, you are a
GEMINI

─────

Ⅱ

Planetary ruler: Mercury

Element: Air

Key phrase: "I think"

Beneficial traits: Lively, adaptable, problem-solver, can see both sides, communicative, intelligent, inquisitive, sense of humor

Challenging traits: Indecisive, needs to control mental activity, superficial, changeable, quick to lose temper, inconsistent moods, unreliable, highly strung nervous system

Body parts: Hands, shoulders, arms, lungs, nerves; prone to respiratory illness and shoulder strain

Essential oils: Lavender, thyme, and eucalyptus can help with respiratory issues; basil, bergamot, pink grapefruit, and ginger are great for soothing the mind; neroli, geranium, and Roman chamomile are generally beneficial

If you were born June 21–July 22, you are a
CANCER

Planetary ruler: Moon

Element: Water

Key phrase: "I feel"

Beneficial traits: Caring, nurturing, mothering, supportive, diplomatic, sustaining, emotional, sensitive, sympathetic, affectionate, intuitive

Challenging traits: Moody, sluggish, can't separate feelings from thoughts, impulsive, overly sensitive, clingy, intense, possessive

Body parts: The breasts and stomach; prone to stomach disorders (including ulcers), heartburn, and water retention

Essential oils: Peppermint, bergamot, and Roman chamomile aid digestion; rosemary and lavender help emotional balance

If you were born July 23–August 22, you are a
LEO

Planetary ruler: Sun

Element: Fire

Key phrase: "I will"

Beneficial traits: Self-confident, warm, generous, faithful, magnetic, enthusiastic, extroverted, loves to entertain, loving, outgoing

Challenging traits: Bossy, dominating, needs to learn delegation, egotistic, possessive, impatient, patronizing

Body parts: Heart, back, spine; prone to back problems

Essential oils: Lemon, rosemary, and ginger for sore backs; rose, marjoram, and melissa for the heart

If you were born August 23–September 22, you are a
VIRGO

Planetary ruler: Mercury

Element: Earth

Key phrase: "I analyze"

Beneficial traits: Intelligent, down-to-earth, discriminatory, detail-oriented, responsible, true friend, loyal, healer, in service to others, shy, homebody, reflective, thoughtful, helpful

Challenging traits: High-strung, perfectionist, overly critical, insecure, skeptical, cold, inflexible

Body parts: Sinuses, respiratory system, bowels; prone to allergies, colds, and flu

Essential oils: Ylang-ylang, Roman chamomile, and melissa are soothing for the overly-taxed mind and feelings of being overwhelmed; ginger, lemon, pink grapefruit, and thyme help with excessive worry and support good health; sandalwood and frankincense alleviate stress and anxiety

If you were born September 23–October 22, you are a
LIBRA

♎

Planetary ruler: Venus

Element: Air

Key phrase: "I balance"

Beneficial traits: Charming, romantic, diplomatic, peace at any price, compassionate, good friend, great lover, even-handed; loves justice, harmony, balance

Challenging traits: Indecisive, uncommitted, people-pleaser, self-centered, lazy, unfocused

Body parts: Lower back, kidneys, ovaries; prone to lower back pain and kidney stones

Essential oils: Geranium and/or fennell for relaxing and assisting the kidneys; basil and/or bergamot for muscle spasms in lower back; black pepper and/or frankincense for nurturing and self-support

If you were born October 23–November 21, you are a
SCORPIO

Planetary ruler: Pluto

Element: Water

Key phrase: "I create"

Beneficial traits: Creative, resourceful, passionate, perceptive, loyal, intense, emotional, deep, sensual, mysterious, driven

Challenging traits: Manipulative, possessive, controlling, cruel, has the sting of a scorpion, unforgiving, strong-willed, needs to learn cooperation and stability in relationships

Body parts: Reproductive and excretory systems; strong body but prone to infections, fevers, and genital problems

Essential oils: Patchouli, ylang-ylang, and neroli are good for the sensual side; sandalwood, clary sage, lavender, and geranium can help ground and soften hard edges; genital support includes melissa, rose, and ginger

If you were born November 22–December 21, you are a
SAGITTARIUS

Planetary ruler: Jupiter

Element: Fire

Key phrase: "I perceive"

Beneficial traits: Philosophical, idealistic, fun-loving, adventurous, freedom-lover, independent, natural entertainer, friendly, has innate understanding of people, forthright, intelligent, excellent communicator

Challenging traits: Impatient, tactless, impulsive, often speaks without thinking, pushy due to extroverted ways, extravagant, impractical, irresponsible

Body parts: Liver, thighs, and hips; sciatica, hip and leg pains, and exhaustion are common problems; prone to stress, tension and addictions

Essential oils: Tea tree, eucalyptus, geranium, and rosemary to support the adventuring nature and free spirit; lavender, neroli, frankincense, and Roman chamomile alleviate tension and stress; basil, juniper, bergamot, black pepper, and ginger help control addictive tendencies

If you were born December 22–January 19, you are a
CAPRICORN

Planetary ruler: Saturn

Element: Earth

Key phrase: "I use"

Beneficial traits: Logical, ambitious, social, hard worker, traditional, strong maternal ties, successful, leader, persistent, loyal friend, sense of humor

Challenging traits: Loner, materialistic, cold, bossy, goal-focused, grudge-bearing, jealous, possessive, dismissive of others' feelings

Body parts: Teeth, bones, kneecaps, and skin; can be prone to sprains, dislocations, skin issues, and TMJ

Essential oils: Eucalyptus, tea tree, ginger, lavender, rosemary, and lemon help with swollen and stiff joints; chamomile, patchouli, sandalwood, and bergamot are anxiety and stress-reducers; strengthening oils are melissa, basil, and peppermint

If you were born January 20–February 18, you are an
AQUARIUS

Planetary ruler: Uranus

Element: Air

Key phrase: "I know"

Beneficial traits: Liberal, idealistic, friendly, kind, people-lovers, humanitarian, futurists, intellectual, original, creative

Challenging traits: Independent, eccentric, impersonal, rebellious, unpredictable, opinionated, fixed, rigid, stubborn, tactless, hates disagreement, needs to be right

Body parts: Circulatory system, shins, and ankles; varicose veins and circulatory problems may be an issue; prone to lower leg and ankle cramps, strains, and breaks

Essential oils: Neroli is the main Aquarius oil; lemon, peppermint, rose, and Roman chamomile are helpful for softening the hard-headedness; cypress, geranium, ginger, eucalyptus, lemon, and neroli assist and stimulate poor circulation.

If you were born February 19–March 20, you are a
PISCES

Planetary ruler: Neptune

Element: Water

Key phrase: "I believe"

Beneficial traits: Psychic, very intuitive, spiritual, sensitive, easy-going dreamers, creative, artistic, vivid imagination, empathetic, compassionate, gentle, kind, patient

Challenging traits: Wishy-washy, lazy, impractical, easily disillusioned, persuadable, moody, depressive

Body parts: Feet, lymphatic system, liver; common ailments are aching feet, bunions, corns, and liver problems.

Essential oils: Black pepper, rosemary, cedarwood, peppermint, bergamot, and basil are great for grounding the dreamy nature; to soothe the inner self use lavender, sandalwood, ravensara, patchouli, rose, ginger, frankincense, and ylang-ylang; tea tree, peppermint, lavender, and lemon help the feet and ankles

Charms, Talismans, and Crystals

Crystals, amulets, talismans, symbols, and other charms may be anointed with the spiritual and healing essential oil of your choice. This is an excellent way to turn a simple, mundane item into an item of magical power and energy.

Birthstones

Select your birthstone from the list below and anoint it with the essential oils for your astrological sign in the above list. If you know your sun sign, moon sign, and rising sign, you can also anoint three stones and carry them with you in a sweet little pouch for round-the-clock support and inspiration. The traditional birthstones according to the American Gem Society are listed by month:

Month:	Stone:
January	Garnet
February	Amethyst
March	Aquamarine
April	Diamond
May	Emerald
June	Pearl
July	Ruby
August	Peridot
September	Sapphire
October	Tourmaline
November	Topaz
December	Tanzanite

Below is a selection of more choices from a spiritually based jeweler, Dyomar Pandan.

ARIES
Main: Bloodstone
Alternate: Diamond
Hindu: Red jasper
Planetary: Jasper
Talismanic: Topaz

TAURUS
Main: Sapphire
Alternate: Amber and rose quartz
Hindu: Rose quartz
Planetary: Aventurine and emerald
Talismanic: Garnet

GEMINI

Main: Agate

Alternate: Chrysophase, citrine, and white sapphire

Hindu: Agate and tourmaline

Planetary: Tiger's eye

Talismanic: Emerald

CANCER

Main: Emerald

Alternate: Moonstone and pearl

Hindu: Moonstone and pearl

Planetary: Moonstone

Talismanic: Sapphire

LEO

Main: Onyx

Alternate: Sardonyx, carnelian, and tourmaline

Hindu: Ruby, Tiger's eye, citrine, and rock crystal

Planetary: Rock crystal

Talismanic: Diamond

VIRGO

Main: Carnelian

Alternate: Jade, jasper, and blue sapphire

Hindu: Carnelian

Planetary: Citrine

Talismanic: Zircon

LIBRA

Main: Peridot

Alternate: Lapis lazuli and opal

Hindu: Opal and aventurine

Planetary: Sapphire

Talismanic: Agate

Scorpio

Main: Aquamarine
Alternate: Beryl, obsidian, and Apache tear
Hindu: Hematite
Planetary: Garnet, ruby, and jasper
Talismanic: Amethyst

Sagittarius

Main: Topaz
Alternate: Turquoise
Hindu: Topaz, turquoise, sodalite, Brazilian agate
Planetary: Topaz
Talismanic: Beryl

Capricorn

Main: Ruby
Alternate: Black onyx
Hindu: Onyx and jet
Planetary: Lapis lazuli
Talismanic: Onyx

Aquarius

Main: Garnet
Alternate: Moss agate and sugilite
Hindu: Garnet
Planetary: Turquoise and lapis lazuli
Talismanic: Jasper

Pisces

Main: Amethyst
Alternate: Aquamarine and rock crystal
Hindu: Amethyst

Planetary: Aquamarine and topaz
Talismanic: Ruby [329]

No matter how you decide to use essential oils in your life, you have abundant avenues to discover what is unique, special, and works for you. These ideas are only a foundation of so many more opportunities to design what speaks to you. You can combine essential oils with religious practices, Pagan or Wiccan traditions, ancient Egyptian or medieval rituals. You can make up your own or use what is provided for you in this book. The more you experiment, the richer the essential oil tradition will become for you. Essential oils have come from the most sacred traditions and civilizations. Become the inventor of your own practices and leave a legacy.

---

329 "Birthstones by Zodiac Sign" kamayojewelry.com/zodiac-signs-birthstones/lucky-stones
-for-zodiac-signs/.

FOURTEEN

My Favorite Essential Oil Recipes

These recipes are designed for adult strength. For children between the ages of five and twelve, dilute to half strength and follow the guidelines in chapter 5.

When you make a blend, a cream, a spray, or any product containing essential oils, please be sure to *label it* correctly and keep away from children.

Essential oils are concentrated, and we want to avoid unsupervised hands spraying the cat or dog with the concoction we have just made.

Treat your products as you would any other chemical mixture, and keep them stored safely away from tiny hands or unsuspecting guests.

Instructions for making inhalers are at the end of this chapter.

Aches and Pains
Muscle Tension Bath

2 drops Roman chamomile essential oil

3 drops vetiver essential oil

4 drops geranium essential oil

Mix with 1 T Epsom salts and add to bath water.

Allergies

Seasonal Allergies (Blend and diffuse)

3 drops lemon essential oil

3 drops clove bud essential oil

2 drops peppermint essential oil

4 drops lavender essential oil

2 drops eucalyptus essential oil

2 drops Roman chamomile essential oil

1–2 drops benzoin essential oil

1 tsp. carrier oil if your diffuser can handle a carrier oil without clogging

Add to diffuser to purify the air. You can also mix this blend in 1 oz. of carrier oil and rub on chest, neck, and under nose for allergy symptom relief.

Do not leave children unattended with this diffusion for more than one minute.

Asthma Relief

The following is a blend that can bring relief to asthma sufferers. Please experiment with the amounts beginning with one drop each, but adding the essential oils that resonate best for your symptoms. This blend will not cure asthma, but may alleviate the symptoms and bring you comfort.

1 DROP EACH OF:

Roman chamomile essential oil, ginger essential oil, frankincense essential oil, benzoin essential oil, geranium essential oil, peppermint essential oil, rose essential oil, lavender essential oil, and marjoram essential oil.

Diffuse this blend for relief. You can also mix it with 1 oz. carrier oil and rub onto chest and neck.

Sinus Relief (Inhaler or cotton ball for sniffing)

5 drops cedarwood essential oil

2 drops peppermint essential oil

2 drops thyme essential oil

3 drops rosemary essential oil

1 drop tea tree essential oil

3 drops ravensara essential oil

5 drops carrier oil

Diffuse this blend for relief if your diffuser can handle a carrier oil without clogging.

Aphrodisiac

2 drops of bergamot essential oil

2 drops rose essential oil

1 drop clary sage essential oil

2 drops ylang-ylang essential oil

1 drop sandalwood essential oil

2 drops geranium essential oil

Diffuse this blend if your diffuser can handle a carrier oil without clogging or mix in 1 oz. carrier oil (fragrant) to use for a couples' massage.

Bruises

Add diluted lavender essential oil to a cold ice compress and place on the bruised area. This constricts the blood vessels and calms the pain and controls swelling. Do not apply ice directly to the skin and do not leave the compress with essential oils on the area for extended periods of time. The rule is fifteen 15 on and 15 minutes off for using an ice compress.

I keep a bag of ice cubes I have frozen with the essential oils or hydrosols right in them. I drop one drop of lavender essential oil into each ice cube tray hole and fill with water. (Use only a tray that is designated for use with essential oils.) When the cubes are frozen, I empty them into a sealable plastic bag, label them as lavender essential oil ice cubes, and keep in the freezer for boo boos and bruises. Be sure to label them well so no one inadvertently uses them in their drinks.

Usually swelling stops in the first 6 to 24 hours. After the swelling has abated, apply the Healing Bruise blend, 1 to 3 drops every few hours, move, and switch between hot and cold compresses using the essential oil blend to increase oxygen to the area and promote healing.

Healing Bruise Blend

3 drops helichrysum essential oil

2 drops tea tree essential oil

3 drops lavender essential oil

2 drops cedarwood essential oil

2 drops lemongrass essential oil

3 drops geranium essential oil

1 drop Roman chamomile essential oil

Mix into 2 tsp. carrier oil like sweet almond, jojoba, or arnica oil. You can also add in 1 oz. aloe vera gel for soothing relief and to alleviate swelling.

Coughs and Colds

For Steam Inhalation

2 C very hot water

6 drops eucalyptus essential oil

6 drops tea tree essential oil

2 drop thyme essential oil

6 drops cedarwood essential oil

3 drops rosemary essential oil

6 drops peppermint essential oil

Mix essential oils into a small bottle. Shake well. Pour hot water into a stainless steel bowl and add 5 drops of the essential oil mixture. Hold your head over the bowl, keep your eyes closed, and drape a towel over your head as you inhale the steam and oils.

Caution: Be careful when inhaling the steam and remember that oftentimes, less is more when using the essential oils.

To Combat a Cold

20 drops orange essential oil

10 drops eucalyptus essential oil

8 drops lemon essential oil

8–10 drops thyme essential oil

6 drops basil essential oil

6 drops palo santo essential oil

4 drops ginger essential oil

Blend all essential oils together and use in a diffuser daily.

Cold Prevention

5 drops lavender essential oil

1 drop peppermint essential oil

5 drops eucalyptus essential oil

3 drops ravensara essential oil

1 drop rosemary essential oil

1 drop tea tree essential oil

Blend and keep in a small dark glass bottle, shake well, and diffuse throughout the cold and flu season. You can add in ½ tsp. carrier oil if you like provided your diffuser doesn't clog with carrier oils. Check the manufacturer's recommendations.

Hand Cleanser (Anti-bacterial, anti-viral, skin nourishing)

1 oz. aloe vera gel

15 drops lavender essential oil

5 drops orange essential oil

2 drops lemon essential oil

Combine in a small portable bottle and carry with you.

Energy

Air Freshener Spritz Blend

TO 12 OZ. OF DISTILLED WATER IN A SPRAY BOTTLE THAT DISPENSES A FINE MIST, ADD:

1 T of vodka or witch hazel

30 drops total of basil, pink grapefruit, lemon,
    orange, rosemary, or ginger essential oils

Shake well and spritz around the room.

Inhaler:

Blend 3 drops of three different essential oils (basil, pink grapefruit, lemon, orange, rosemary, peppermint, dill, black pepper, or ginger essential oils) in 1 tsp. carrier oil and create an inhaler. Use when you feel a need for a burst of energy.

Palm Method:

Any single diluted essential oil—basil, pink grapefruit, lemon, orange, rosemary, thyme, peppermint, or ginger essential oil—can be applied to your palms, one drop at a time. Rub hands together, cup your palms, and inhale for a quick pick-me-up.

Household Cleaners

#1 All-Purpose Household Spray
(cleans, kills bacteria, deodorizes, and freshens)

INTO 1 QUART WATER, MIX:

2 drops rosemary essential oil

4 drops lemon essential oil

3 drops eucalyptus essential oil

4 drops lavender essential oil

2 drops thyme or tea tree essential oil

1 tsp. vodka or witch hazel to be a dispersant as
    the essential oils will separate from the water

Shake well and pour into a spray bottle. Be sure to shake before each use.

#2 Recipe for Household Cleaner

INTO 1 QUART WATER, MIX:

 3–4 drops lavender essential oil

 5–6 drops rosemary or thyme essential oil

2 drops lemon essential oil

1 tsp. vodka or witch hazel for dispersant

Shake well and pour into a spray bottle. Be sure to shake before each use as the essential oils will separate from the water.

Recipe for Window/Glass Cleaner
(For windows and stainless steel)
IN A SPRAY BOTTLE, MIX TOGETHER:

50 percent water

50 percent vinegar (white)

10 to 12 drops lemon essential oil

Shake well and use on windows for a clean shine. Because there are not chemicals in this mixture, you may have to rub a bit longer to allow the water to evaporate. It's worth the extra time to save yourself and your environment from alcohol and chemical airborne residue.

Insect Repellant

Nontopical Insect Repellant Spray
POUR INGREDIENTS INTO A SPRAY BOTTLE. SHAKE WELL BEFORE USING.

15 drops lavender essential oil

10 drops eucalyptus essential oil

10 drops tea tree essential oil

6 drops vetiver essential oil

6 drops bergamot essential oil

2 drops basil essential oil

2 oz. distilled water

2 oz. white vinegar

This blend is meant to be diffused and spritzed into the air around you to ward off insects and is not to be used directly on the skin or internally.

Insomnia

2 drops ylang-ylang essential oil

2 drops lavender essential oil

2 drops marjoram essential oil

2 drops clary sage essential oil

1 drop Roman chamomile essential oil

1 drop dill essential oil

1 oz. spring water

Combine in a small spray bottle and spray on your pillow before bed for better sleep.

Meditation and Spirituality (For use in a diffuser)
Grounding
Sandalwood, patchouli, frankincense, bergamot, vetiver, myrrh

Enlightening
Helichrysum, rose, ylang-ylang, melissa, myrrh, palo santo, pink grapefruit

Calming
Lavender, sandalwood, neroli, frankincense, ylang-ylang, clary sage

Relaxation and Stress Relief
Bath (relaxing, soothing)
3 drops lavender essential oil

3 drops ylang-ylang essential oil

2 drops bergamot essential oil

2 drops rose or geranium essential oil

Mix with 1 T of Epsom salts and add to bath water

Bath (to reduce anxiety)
3 drops vetiver essential oil

2 drops cedarwood essential oil

1 drop palo santo essential oil

2 drops frankincense essential oil

Mix with 1 T of Epsom salts and add to bath water

Inhaler (or sniff from a cotton ball soaked in mixture below)
3 drops ylang-ylang essential oil

6 drops vetiver essential oil

6 drops lavender essential oil

Skin and Face Creams

I like to use (organic) apricot oil, sweet almond oil, argan oil, carrot seed oil, geranium oil, pomegranate seed oil, and rose hip seed oil as carrier oils to mix with my essential oils.

When you make creams and lotions you may want to have a separate set of measuring cups, measuring spoons, and stirring spoons designated for this purpose. This keeps your essential oil utensils clean and bacteria free and your everyday kitchen utensils untouched by oils, waxes, and hydrosols. I also recommend using a separate blender for making face creams and lotions.

Acne

There are basically two essential oils that can help spot-treat pimples and blemishes: tea tree and lavender essential oils. Dilute them and then apply to breakouts. Rotate them every other day and use for three days, then take two days off and begin again until blemishes subside. (Perform a patch test first before applying to skin as you may be super sensitive to these essential oils.)

First, wash, and cleanse your face. Place a drop of either diluted lavender or tea tree essential oil on a cotton swab and dab it gently on the pimple or breakout. Rotate the essential oils used. Apply three days in a row, then take two days off and you can begin again. (This could take two to three weeks for you to see results.)

Other effective anti-acne essential oils are bergamot, benzoin, Roman chamomile, yarrow, helichrysum, thyme, lemongrass, cinnamon, cedarwood, geranium, pink grapefruit, lemon, lemongrass, orange, patchouli, peppermint, rosemary, sandalwood, vetiver, and ylang-ylang. These should be diluted in a carrier oil (half and half) and applied carefully to your skin. It's a good idea to do a skin patch test before using these oils.

Dry skin face cream

Use 50 ml or 1.75 oz. of base cream or lotion
2 drops ylang-ylang essential oil
3 drops geranium essential oil
3 drops neroli essential oil
2 drops yarrow essential oil

2 drop rose essential oil

3 drops orange essential oil

Blend together.

Itching

10 drops Roman chamomile essential oil

10 drops lavender essential oil

5 drops frankincense essential oil

5 drops sandalwood essential oil

Mix with 20 oz. water or 2 T sweet almond oil. Spray on skin or massage in as needed.

Scars

2 drops lavender essential oil

1 drop rosemary essential oil

1 drop helichrysum essential oil

1 tsp. jojoba, sweet almond, or rose hip carrier oil

Apply to scar two to four times a day. Lightly tap on the scar tissue to encourage healing.

Difficult scars

5 drops helischrysum essential oil

5 drops lavender essential oil

2 drops myrrh essential oil

2 drops thyme essential oil

2 drops frankincense essential oil

½ tsp. argan or hazelnut oil

½ tsp. wheat germ oil

1 tsp. jojoba oil

Mix together and apply on tough scars three times per day for six weeks.

Essential oils that help scars heal are: lavender, basil, helichrysum, frankincense, rosemary, neroli, thyme, myrrh, and yarrow.

Wrinkles

Age Arrester Serum

(Makes about 3 oz. and should keep for nine months up to a year.)

6 tsp. apricot kernel oil

5 tsp. rosehip seed oil

4 tsp. evening primrose oil

3 tsp. pomegranate oil

2 tsp. borage oil

1 tsp. vitamin E oil

5 drops rosemary essential oil

4 drops helichrysum essential oil

4 drops lavender essential oil

4 drops frankincense essential oil

3 drops geranium essential oil

4 drops rose essential oil

1 drop lemon essential oil

Mix together and store in sterilized 1 or 2 oz. dropper bottles. Keep extras in the refrigerator until ready to use. Apply gently and use every night for age-defying results.

Firming Face Serum

2 T avocado, grapeseed, or pomegranate carrier oil

8 drops cedarwood essential oil

7 drops geranium essential oil

3 drops frankincense essential oil

3 drops myrrh essential oil

2 drops neroli essential oil

1 drop lavender essential oil

Combine, mix well, and place in a dropper bottle. Label it and use twice a day, morning and night, to keep face skin firm and young.

Face Cream

(Make it yourself! Lasts for up to a year refrigerated; makes a great gift!)

I call this my WOW Cream

1 T apricot kernel oil

1 T wheat germ oil

2 tsp. jojoba oil

1 tsp. evening primrose oil

1 tsp. borage oil

½ tsp. carrot seed oil

½ tsp. vitamin E oil

10 drops yarrow essential oil

8 drops helichrysum essential oil

8 drops benzoin essential oil

3 drops rose essential oil

2 drops vetiver essential oil

2 drops patchouli essential oil

2 drops neroli essential oil

2 drops lavender essential oil

2 drops lemongrass essential oil

2–4 drops of your favorite essential oil for aroma

½ tsp. vodka or vanilla extract

1 T fractionated coconut oil

¼ C cacao butter

3 T shea butter

1 T beeswax

¼ C aloe vera gel

⅔ C rose hydrosol

BEFORE YOU BEGIN:

You will need to have dark glass face cream jars on hand that you pre-sterilize and cool. Also create labels for your jars at this time.

Sterilize your blender with boiling hot water and allow to dry.

Use a double boiler, or devise a way to melt ingredients over hot water bath.

STEPS:

1. Sterilize your containers and have them ready and dry.

2. Combine essential oils, vitamin E, and vodka in a small glass container and set aside.

3. Melt cacao butter, shea butter, beeswax, and coconut oil together in a double boiler or pan over hot water in a saucepan.

4. Allow the mixture to cool a bit, then add to sterilized blender with almond, wheat germ, and jojoba oils. Blend on low.

5. Stream in hydrosol and aloe vera gel while on low blend. Blend for a few minutes until mixture become thick.

6. Pour in essential oil mixture and blend very well (about 2 to 3 minutes) until all are completely mixed in.

7. Pour into dry jars and allow mixture to cool before putting the lid on. Add labels.

8. Store extra jars in the refrigerator until use. (The first time I made this blend it had a grainy feeling. You can let a dollop of it sit in your palm and your body heat will soften the mixture. The second time I made it, I blended it for a longer time and it came out smooth, not grainy.) Men and women can use this WOW Cream at night or in the morning.

Dry Skin Face Cream

Use 50 ml or 1.75 oz. of prepared base cream or lotion

2 drops ylang-ylang essential oil

3 drops geranium essential oil

3 drops neroli essential oil

2 drops palma rosa essential oil

3 drops orange essential oil

Blend together.

Face
Essential Oil Moisturizing Mask
1 oz. coconut, avocado, pomegranate, argan, or sweet almond oil

5 drops geranium essential oil

5 drops lavender essential oil

2 drops frankincense essential oil

1 drop helichrysum essential oil

2 drops sandalwood essential oil

1 drop patchouli essential oil

Mix together and store in a dark glass bottle with a stopper or dropper. Shake well before using. Pour a small dime-size dollop into your hand and massage over your entire face. Leave on for 20 to 30 minutes (this is a good time to meditate or relax with soft music) and then wash off. Gently pat dry your face and apply a daytime face cream of your choosing.

Fast Version of Moisturizing Mask
1 T sweet almond oil

1 drop rose essential oil

1 drop pink grapefruit essential oil

Mix well and apply to face. Leave on for 20–30 minutes then pat off. Apply Day Wear for Face (see next recipe) under makeup or use without makeup.

Day Wear for Face
⅞ oz. apricot kernel oil or carrot seed oil

1 drop frankincense essential oil

2 drops lavender essential oil

1 drop pink grapefruit essential oil

1 drop helichrysum essential oil

1 drop vetiver or lemongrass essential oil

Mix in a 1 oz. dark glass bottle with lid or stopper.

Shake vigorously to mix oils together. (Be sure to shake well before each use.) From the bottle, drop a few drops into the palms of your hands and gently apply to face. Allow oils to soak in for 5 minutes, then apply makeup.

Night Cream for Face

⅞ oz. apricot kernel oil, pomegranate, or carrot seed oil

1 drop frankincense essential oil

2 drops lavender essential oil

1 drop pink grapefruit essential oil

1 drop helichrysum essential oil

1 drop vetiver or lemongrass essential oil

Mix in a 1 oz. dark glass bottle with dropper/stopper.

Shake to mix (shake before each use) and drop a few drops into palm and rub onto face. Allow to soak in for 5 minutes before going to bed.

Wounds

If the wound is fresh, disinfect the area with 2 C of warm water mixed with 5 drops of lavender and 2 to 3 drops of tea tree essential oils.

Apply 2–3 drops of lavender essential oil blended with 6 drops of carrier oil to bandage material and place over wound. Be sure to change this dressing once or twice a day using the essential oils mix. When the wound is sufficiently healed—about three to four days—you can leave it uncovered. Or recover if more time is needed.

If the wound or cut requires stitches, consult your doctor and make sure he or she has no objection to using lavender essential oil, diluted on the wound. Some medical professionals prefer to hold off on essential oils application until the sutures are removed.

Weight Loss
Cellulite Control Rub
COMBINE:

10 drops pink grapefruit essential oil

5 drops rosemary essential oil

2 drops each peppermint, black pepper, and ginger essential oils

Blend with 1 T of carrier oil before applying to the body.

One Appetite Suppression (Blend for a diffuser or an inhaler)
MIX TOGETHER:

40 drops orange essential oil

20 drops lemon essential oil

12 drops ginger essential oil

12 drops peppermint essential oil

6 drops thyme essential oil

Add a few drops of this blend to your diffuser 20 minutes before meals.

If you can't diffuse at work, make yourself an inhaler and carry it with you. Use inhaler 20 to 30 minutes before meals.

Two Appetite Suppression (Blend for a diffuser or an inhaler)

10 drops neroli essential oil

5 drops ginger essential oil

5 drops pink grapefruit essential oil

5 drops cinnamon essential oil

6 drops thyme essential oil

2 drops black pepper essential oil

Add a few drops to your diffuser and/or inhaler and use 20 to 30 minutes before meals.

How to Make an Inhaler

You will need to buy some blank inhalers. Look for the ones that are made with organic cotton wicks and not ones that are over-processed and bleached. The inhaler will have three parts: the exterior tube-like case, the plug at the bottom, and the cotton wick inside.

Next, follow one of two methods for making the inhaler. The use of a small amount of carrier oil is important so the essential oils are diluted. I use about half a teaspoon of carrier oil for each essential oil blend I make.

1. Mix/blend the essential oils and carrier oil in a small ceramic ramekin or a clean glass container and soak the wick in the blend for an hour or so. Cover with a lid or plastic wrap while soaking to prevent evaporation. Essential oils may eat the plastic, so make sure the plastic wrap does not touch the mixture. When soaked thoroughly, lift wick out with a tweezer and place inside the tube, snapping the end on the bottom. Screw the outer tube case onto the inhaler and you're done.

2. Drop the diluted essential oil mixture onto the wick one drop at a time until the wick is soaked through. This is tedious because of the size of the wick and also challenging to manage because the oils come out quickly. If you choose this method, follow the same directions for finishing the inhaler as in the first.

Your inhaler is portable, and you can use it as frequently as you need to for any number of benefits ranging from cold and flu protection to meditation and enlightenment.

How to Make a Roller Ball

Purchase some blank roller ball applicator bottles/tubes for essential oils. Choose the essential oils that will assist your healing or alleviate your complaint. Lift or screw the roller ball off the top of the tube/bottle.

Pour 1 tsp. of a carrier oil (you have your choice of many mentioned in this book) into the roller ball applicator/bottle and add to it the drops of the essential oils you want to use. Make sure your dilution is 60/40 carrier oils to essential oils. Snap the roller ball back onto the tube/bottle. Shake well.

Apply this mixture to your feet, hands, sore points, or wherever you want relief per the blend you selected.

A nighttime roller ball application, as you are going to bed, helps the body heal during the night.

There are many recipes available in books and on the Internet. I encourage you to experiment, play, and be willing to make a few blends that don't quite work for you. One big hint is to get yourself a stack of 3x5" index cards and make notes on them for the blends you create.

Nothing is more frustrating than when you come up with a blend that knocks your socks off but you can't remember which oils and what amounts you used because the phone rang just as you were adding the last drop and you lost your train of thought.

Your notes will not only help you remember that fantastic blend you created, but will also allow you to extrapolate from a base blend and continue creating more and more fabulous products for yourself and your family.

I hope you have enjoyed this journey with me. I have a really good feeling that this is a great beginning for your new life with natural products and alternative healing techniques. May your life be filled with these amazing essential oils and magnificent aromas.

Final Thoughts

You made it! Congratulations on making the journey through fifty essential oils and absolutes. There are many more essential oils available in this abundant natural world of ours. The count is well over one hundred in circulation today. Maybe we can continue our expedition and the next fifty will make up Volume Two.

Essential oils do more than just smell good. They heal us on several levels. Many rural civilizations in third-world countries are farming plants and trees that produce essential oils and are turning their economies around using sustainable practices without pesticides.

Researchers across the globe are experimenting with essential oils and clinically testing the results of healing claims and chemical properties. Progress is being made in laboratories around the world as scientists delve into their origin and elements.

Healers from a variety of disciplines are using vibrational energy to bring about a shift for the better in people suffering from conditions and illnesses. Essential oils play a big part in holistic treatment and integrated medicine practices. It's all coming together. Healing practices are beginning to overlap and share. What seemed to be on the fringe decades ago is now becoming mainstream.

Football teams are meditating before games. Even police forces in Canada meditate before they go on patrol. Yoga studios are on every corner and good health and sound nutrition are becoming inextricably linked in the public's mind. Even firefighters are turning to vegan fare for their meals in fire houses.

We are using ancient knowledge in this age of information to help ourselves and the planet. It's a very good time to be alive.

Whether you become a casual user of essential oils, or if you go further and become a professional practitioner or Aromatherapist, you will be rubbing elbows with some of the smartest natural physicians in history.

Next time you need a remedy, watch to see what you do. Will you come off automatic and look for an essential oil to provide some relief, or will you reach for a pharmaceutical? You'll know exactly what to do that best serves your needs.

As the worlds of standard medicine, integrative medicine, and alternative therapies move closer and closer together you'll find yourself perched on the cutting edge of this emerging field. It is where the future is headed.

As science investigates more about the properties and results of using essential oils, natural healing will become more prominent for the savvy. Having read this book, you're already in the top percentile and ahead of the game.

We can all join the healing parade and use ancient knowledge combined with today's science for a happier and healthier tomorrow. The future is around the bend and the merger will happen in our lifetime.

Glossary

Analgesic: Pain relieving

Antiallergenic: Reduces symptoms of allergies

Antibacterial: Fights bacterial growth

Antiblastic: Prevents growth of a parasite

Anticancerous: Inhibits growth of cancer cells

Anticonvulsant: Helps control convulsions

Antidepressant: Helps to counteract depression and lifts the mood

Antifungal: Prevents the growth of fungi

Anti-inflammatory: Reduces inflammation

Antimicrobial: Reduces or resists microbes

Antiphlogistic: Counteracts inflammation

Antipyretic: Reduces fever

Antirheumatic: Helps to combat rheumatism

Antiseborrheic: Fights a skin condition that causes scaly patches and red skin, mainly on the scalp

Antiseptic: Helps control infection

Antispasmodic: Helps to control spasms

Antitumoral: Inhibits the development of tumors

Antitussive: Relieves coughing

Antiviral: Counteracts the effects of viruses

Aperitif: Stimulates the appetite

Aphrodisiac: Increases sexual desire and sexual functioning

Aromatic: Having a pleasant and distinctive smell

Astringent: Causes skin tissue to contract; good for toning skin

Autoimmune support: A disease in which the body's immune system attacks healthy cells

Bactericide: Destroys bacteria

Cardiotonic: Exerting a favorable, so-called tonic effect on the action of the heart

Carminative: Settles the digestive system and relieves flatulence

Cephalic: Stimulating and clearing the mind

Cholagogue: Promotes the secretion of bile into the duodenum

Cicatrisant: Promotes healing by scar tissue formation

Cordial: A heart tonic

Cytophylactic: Increases the leukocyte activity to defend the body against infection

Deodorant: Works against and masks body odor

Depurative: Helps to detoxify and to combat impurities in the blood and body

Detoxifier: Combats impurities in the blood and body

Diaphoretic: Helps to promote perspiration

Digestive: Helps digestion

Disinfectant: Causes the destruction of bacteria

Diuretic: Helps increase the production of urine

Emenagogue: Promotes and stimulates menstrual flow

Emollient: Softening and soothing to the skin

Euphoric: Feeling intense excitement and happiness

Expectorant: Helps to expel mucus from the lungs

Febrifuge: Helps to combat fever

Fungicidal: Inhibiting the growth of fungi

Fungicide: Destroys fungal infections

Haemostatic: Retarding or stopping bleeding

Hemostatic: Arresting hemorrhage, styptic

Hepatic: A tonic for the liver

Hypotensive: Lowers blood pressure

Immune stimulant: Induces activation or increases activity of any of the components of the immune system

Laxative: Helps with bowel movements

Lymphatic stimulant: Promotes lymph flow, which in turn removes waste products

Memory enhancer: Promotes better memory recall

Metabolic stimulant: Boosts the rate at which body processes function

Nervine: Strengthens and tones the nerves and nervous system

Parasiticide: Kills parasites (especially those other than bacteria or fungi)

Rubefacient: Causes redness of the skin by stimulating blood circulation

Relaxant: Promotes relaxation or reduces tension

Restorative: Restores health, strength, or a feeling of well-being

Reviving: Gives new strength or energy

Sedative: Provides a soothing and calming effect

Skin tonic: Tones, stimulates, or freshens the skin

Stimulant: Provides an invigorating action on the body and circulation

Stomach tonic: Helps digestion and improves appetite

Stomachic: Promotes the appetite or assists digestion

Styptic: Capable of stopping bleeding when applied to a wound

Sudorific: Induces sweating

Tonic: Gives a feeling of vigor or well-being; invigorating

Uterine: Relating to the uterus or womb

Uterine agent: Induces contraction or greater tonicity of the uterus

Vasodilator: Causes vasodilatation, the dilatation of blood vessels

Vermifuge: Expels intestinal worms

Vulnerary: Helps to heal wounds and sores and helps to prevent tissue degeneration

Sources

Internet

3wisemenessentials.com/essential_oils.html from www.anandaapothecary.com
/aromatherapy-essential-oils/organicpatchouli.html

aromatherapy-cypress.blogspot.com/

articles.mercola.com/herbal-oils/eucalyptus-oil.aspx

articles.mercola.com/herbal-oils/thyme-oil.aspx

Ashi Aromatics Inc., www.ashitherapy.com

beforeitsnews.com/self-sufficiency/2015/06/23-awesome-uses-for-lemongrass
-essential-oil-2491270.html

community.fortunecity.ws/roswell/chaney/191/id103.htm

community.fortunecity.ws/roswell/chaney/191/id119.htm from thehealthy
havenblog.com/tag/oils/

Deomar Pandan Jewelry, http://kamayojewelry.com/zodiac-signs-birthstones
/lucky-stones-for-zodiac-signs/

Essential oils and Animals: www.holisticanimalassociation.com

fitlife.tv/thyme-oil-a-natural-antibiotic/

www.newagearticles.com/Article/Counterculture-Aromatherapy—Patchouli
-Essential-Oil/98

Holistic Animal Association, www.holisticanimalassociation.com

www.jonnsaromatherapy.com/pdf/Briggs_Real_Story_of_Gary_Young_2013.pdf

en.wikipedia.org/wiki/Anointing

www.slideshare.net/herbalista/alternative-medicine-aromatherapy-essential-oils
-balms-and-lotions-copia

uk.pinterest.com/pin/64880050857509472/

www.botanical.com/botanical/mgmh/s/sages-05.html

www.lewrockwell.com/2014/04/gaye-levy/33—uses-for-essential-lemon-oil/

www.yellowstaressentials.wordpress.com/profiles-of-essential-oils/from
/insomnia/entangledbotanicalsbyashleynovember.com/tag/essential-oils
-and-flower-essences/

mothernaturesgoodies.blogspot.com/2013/08/how-to-use-frankincense-oil.html

newresearchfindingstwo.blogspot.com/2015/08/eucalyptus-oil-essential-oil.html

newresearchfindingstwo.blogspot.com/2015/08/thyme-oil-natural-antibiotic.html

Pregnancy: www.naha.org/assets/uploads/PregnancyGuidelines-Oct11.pdf

stores.ebay.com/Anabells-Escentials/The-Essentials-of-Essential-Oils.html

thearomablog.com/category/essential-oil-profile/page/5/

wildedibleandmedicinalplants.blogspot.com/2010_07_01_archive.html

wongwhs.pbworks.com/w/file/fetch/91644000/SpiceTrade.docx

www.ahimsacenter.com.au/product/essential-oil/

http://www.anandaapothecary.com/aromatherapy-essential-oils-news/2005/10
/patchouli-oil-counterculture-scent.html.

www.aromarakesh.com/Essential.html

www.aromaweb.com/essentialoils/essentialoilsforsummer.asp

www.astridestella.info/p/holistic-therapies.html

www.ayurvedicoils.com/tag/ayurv

www.backdoorsurvival.com/33—awesome-uses-of-lemon-essential-oil/

www.barnesandnoble.com/w/the-new-age-herbalist-anne-mc-intyre/1113128930

www.beautyhealthsupply.com/essential.htm

beforeitsnews.com/self-sufficiency/2014/04/33-awesome-uses-of-lemon-essential
-oil-2473562.html.

www.biosourcenaturals.com/essential-oils-for-circulation-hair-growth.htm

www.biosourcenaturals.com/essential-oils-for-sinuses.htm

www.boatloadsofhealth.com/posts/benefits-of-spikenard-essential-oil/the
aromablog.com/tag/chemistry

www.consciouslifenews.com/eucalyptus-essential-oil-extraordinaire/1174549/

www.cryofoods.com/spice-for-life-encyclopedia.asp

www.daily-survival.blogspot.com/feeds/posts/default?orderby=updated

www.deancoleman.org/essentialref.htm

www.dreamingearth.com/blog/rosemary-essential-oil-part-two/

www.essential-aromatherapy-oils.com/Patchouly-Essential-Oil.html

www.essentialoilroundtable.com/kelly-azzaro/

www.fda.gov/Cosmetics/ProductsIngredients/Products/ucm127054.htm

www.fragrantessence.com/msg8.htm

www.gleneals.blogspot.no/

www.goldensnaturals.com/blogs/essential-oils-what-are-they

www.healthwizardry.com/magickal-oils/

www.incensewarehouse.com/Patchoulis-History-and-Use_ep_25–1.html

www.itmamsterdam.blogspot.com/2015_10_01_archive

www.moondragon.org/aromatherapy/aromatherapyoils/cedarwoodoil.html

www.moondragon.org/aromatherapy/aromatherapyoils/lemonoil.html

www.moondragon.org/aromatherapy/aromatherapyoils/ylangylangoil.html

www.naha.org/assets/uploads/Animal_Aromatherapy_Safety_NAHA.pdf www
.elertgadget.com/palert/aromatherapy_favorites_patchouli_essential_oil_6250
.htm

www.naringol.com/herbals_en.php

www.naturalblaze.com/2014/04/33–awesome-uses-of-lemon-essential-oil.html

www.naturalblaze.com/2015/06/23–awesome-uses-for-lemongrass.html

www.healthy-holistic-living.com/thyme-oil-natural-antibiotic.html

www.articlesfactory.com/articles/health/ … y-favorites-patchouli-essential-oil

www.natural-skin-care-info.com/patchouli-oil.html

www.occultlectures.com/properties-of-essential-oils.html

www.parasitetesting.co.uk/wiki/remedies

www.pinemeadowsblog.blogspot.com/2015/01/roller-ball-essential-oil-recipes.html

www.puressentialoils.co.za/newsletters.htm

www.refreshingnews99.blogspot.com/2015/08/spiritual-and-magical-properties-
of.html https://quizlet.com/25033568/essential-oils-1–49–hebs-50–till-end-
flash-cards/

www.spafromscratch.com/three-awesome-frankincense-essential-oil-recipes/

www.spiritvoyage.com/blog/index.php/aromatherapy-and-yoga-everyday
-essential-oils/

www.static.premiersite.co.uk/20141/docs/6214211_2.pdf

www.thearomablog.com/a-sacred-and-spiritual-scent-palo-santo/

www.theraindropfairy.weebly.com/essential-oils.html

www.thesavvyoiler.com/top-12–spring-essential-oil-diffuser-recipes/

www.thesavvyoiler.com/top-12–spring-essential-oil-diffuser-recipes/

www.thesleuthjournal.com/33–awesome-uses-lemon-essential-oil/

wakeup-world.com/2014/04/21/33-awesome-uses-of-lemon-essential-oil
-for-home-and-health/

www.wiccazone.net/magical_herbal_enclyclopedia_l.htm

www.wikipediadiet.com/2015/10/how-to-use-eucalyptus-essential-oil.html

www.willowtreewisdom.com/thyme-honey/

www.ylessentialoils.com/7Oils_100Solutions.pdf

zenrosegarden.com/essential-oils.html

Books

(var.) A Modern Herbal: How to Grow, Cook and Use Herbs. London: Treasure Press, 1974.

Baker, Jerry. *Supermarket Super Gardens.* Wixom, MI: American Master Products, 2008.

Becker, Robert, and Gary Selden. *The Body Electric: Electromagnetism and the Foundation of Life.* New York: William Morrow Paperbacks First Edition, 1985.

Borino, Bob. *Herbal Remedies.* Boca Raton, FL: Globe Communications, 1983.

Chardenon, Ludo. *In Praise of Wild Herbs.* Santa Barbara, CA: Capra Press, 1984.

Cooper, Guy, and Gordon Taylor. *A Multitude of Mints.* Macclesfield, UK: Herb Society/Juniper Press, 1981.

———. *The Romance of Rosemary.* Macclesfield, UK: Herb Society/Juniper Press, 1981.

Crow, David. *Sacred Smoke: The Magic and Medicine of Palo Santo.* Kindle Edition.

Cunningham, Scott. *Encyclopedia of Magical Herbs.* Woodbury, MN: Llewelyn Publications, 2013, second edition.

Garland, Sarah. *The Complete Book of Herbs and Spices.* London: Frances Lincoln Limited, 1979.

Harris, Ben Charles. *The Compleat Herbal.* New York: Larchmont Books, 1972.

Jarmey, Chris, and John Tindall. *Acupressure for Common Ailments.* New York: Simon and Schuster, 1991.

Linden, Stanton J., ed. *The Alchemy Reader: from Hermes Trismegistus to Isaac Newton.* New York: Cambridge University Press, 2003.

Lucas, Richard. *Nature's Medicines.* New York: Award Books, 1966.

Morris, Marlene, and Kac Young. *Star Power: 12 Days That Can Change Your Life.* Los Angeles: Marlene Morris Ministries, 2006.

(var.) Mysteries of the Unknown. Alexandria VA: Time Life Books Series, 1988.

Petulengro, Leon. *Herbs, Health and Astrology.* Boca Raton, FL: Globe Communications, 1996.

Reichstein, Gail. *Wood Becomes Water: Chinese Medicine in Everyday Life.* New York: Kodansha America, 1998.

Schiller, Carol, and David Schiller. *500 Formulas for Aromatherapy: Mixing Essential Oils for Every Use.* New York: Sterling Publishing, 1994.

Schnaubelt, Kurt. *The Healing Intelligence of Essential Oils.* Rochester, VT: Healing Arts Press, 2011.

Tisserand, Robert, and Rodney Young. *Essential Oil Safety: A Guide for Health Care Professionals.* London: Churchill Livingstone, 2002.

Tourles, Stephanie. *Organic Body Care Recipes.* North Adams, MA: Storey Publishing, 2007.

Wade, Carlson. *Folk Remedies.* Boca Raton, FL, Globe Communications, 1988.

Weil, Andrew. *Health and Healing: The Philosophy of Integrative Medicine and Optimum Health.* Boston: Houghton Mifflin, 1988.

Williams, Jude C. *Jude's Herbal Home Remedies.* St. Paul, MN: Llewelyn Publications, 1996.

Williams, Tom. *The Complete Illustrated Guide to Chinese Medicine.* New York: Barnes and Noble, 1996.

Worwood, Valerie Ann. *The Complete Book of Essential Oils and Aromatherapy.* Novato, CA: New World Library, 1991.

Young, Kac. *Feng Shui… The Easy Way.* Los Angeles: Marlene Morris Ministries, 2007.

———. *Supreme Healing.* Los Angeles, Marlene Morris Ministries, 2010.

Index

evening primrose, 51, 341, 342

exhaustion, 68, 108, 126, 130, 138, 152, 163, 184, 221, 324

expectorant, 64, 70, 84, 86, 95, 106, 135, 145, 154, 162, 166, 191, 195, 200, 245, 353

extreme unction, 285

facial, 104, 109, 112, 143, 173

farming, 35, 237, 349

fatigue, 60, 61, 89, 106, 109, 154, 155, 163, 179, 180, 184, 196, 198, 213, 221, 257, 266, 309, 314, 316

FDA, 37

fear, 21, 79, 80, 114, 119, 121, 157, 158, 256–258, 267

febrifuge, 79, 126, 176, 210, 353

fennel, 42, 53, 288

fertility, 142, 175

fetotoxicity, 50

fever, 61, 62, 74, 80, 81, 83, 86, 88, 91, 93, 111, 123, 168, 210, 212, 217, 351, 353

fidelity, 157, 190

fir, 11, 42

flatulence, 91, 128, 136, 182, 205, 316, 352

flu, 22, 76, 126, 141, 142, 168, 196, 197, 208, 219, 231, 322, 335, 347

focus, 67, 70, 83, 84, 103, 155, 194, 199, 201, 255

forgiveness, 180, 190, 199, 255, 258, 268

fractionated coconut oil, 51, 202, 203, 342

frangipani, 31, 234, 238, 239, 247

frankincense, 11–13, 30, 53, 72, 81, 82, 89, 95–100, 105, 114, 119, 120, 129, 132, 134, 140, 144, 148, 151, 161, 164, 169, 179, 190, 191, 194, 197, 199, 203, 209, 216, 218, 219, 224, 230, 231, 236, 242, 248, 257–259, 261, 263, 265–268, 270–274, 279, 280, 282, 283, 302, 305, 313, 319, 322–324, 326, 332, 338, 340, 341, 344, 345

Friedmann, Terry, 201

fungus, 64, 76, 205

galbanum, 11, 288

gall bladder, 123, 131

Ganot, Lucien, 151

gargle, 74, 174, 184

garlic, 43, 97

Garnier, 111

gas, 9, 13, 91, 128, 136, 143, 226, 228

Gemini, 320, 328

geranium, 30, 53, 63, 67, 72, 78, 81, 82, 85, 94, 100, 105, 113, 119, 120, 125, 131, 134, 140, 148, 152, 157, 161, 171–176, 180, 185, 190, 199, 203, 214, 222, 224, 236, 242, 244, 248, 250, 257–259, 266, 269, 271, 272, 281, 283, 284, 293, 303, 304, 311, 315, 317, 320, 323–325, 331–334, 338, 339, 341, 343, 344

ginger, 4, 30, 33, 42, 53, 90, 120, 129, 135–140, 143, 144, 148, 152, 168, 185, 190, 199, 208, 209, 213, 214, 224, 231, 238, 239, 251, 257–259, 264, 270, 278, 303, 310, 311, 313, 320, 322–326, 332, 335, 336, 346

gout, 68, 106, 150, 187, 215, 231, 316

grapefruit, 30, 42, 52, 63, 71, 85, 90, 94, 138, 139, 144, 148, 152, 156, 175, 180, 185, 199, 203, 209, 214, 218, 220–225, 228, 231, 239, 244, 247, 251, 257–259, 262, 265, 266, 270, 272, 277, 278, 282–284, 303, 320, 322, 335, 336, 338, 339, 344–346

grapeseed, 51, 200, 341

inhalation, 19, 54, 93, 109, 174, 197, 200, 201, 216, 221, 223, 224, 334

inhaler, 48, 71, 81, 84, 104, 143, 318, 332, 336, 338, 346, 347

inner child, 258, 274

insects, 62, 66, 89, 100, 104, 109, 118, 145, 149, 173, 200–202, 212, 217, 337

insecurity, 111, 258, 273

insomnia, 60, 77, 91, 111, 131, 141, 150–152, 158, 160, 163, 166, 174, 186–188, 212, 216, 220, 226, 240, 249, 251, 258, 275, 309, 310, 337

irritability, 104, 151, 160, 177, 187

irritation, 39, 50, 55, 66, 67, 78, 129, 130, 169, 172, 185, 194, 209, 229, 251, 258, 276

itching, 61, 66, 168, 340

Jaborandi, 43

jasmine, 31, 53, 112, 159, 234, 235, 247, 248, 257–259, 304

jealousy, 111, 259, 276, 302, 311

joint pain, 200, 212

jojoba, 51, 77, 88, 100, 113, 143, 144, 179, 200, 209, 218, 245, 260, 334, 340, 342, 343

joy, 21, 33, 119, 140, 162, 237, 259, 277, 290, 292, 295–297, 306, 310

juniper, 11, 42, 53, 190, 202, 231, 288, 324

Juniperus virginia, 200

Keller, Helen, 18

khas-khas, 150

laurel leaf, 42

lavender, 8, 13–15, 17, 30, 33, 38, 53, 59–63, 67, 69, 72, 75, 78, 81, 84, 85, 89, 90, 93, 94, 99, 100, 105, 110, 113, 114, 124, 125, 129, 132–134, 138, 143, 144, 147, 148, 151, 152, 156, 157, 159, 161, 164, 165, 169, 173, 175, 179, 180, 185, 187,

188, 190, 194, 198–201, 203, 209, 212, 214, 218, 224, 230, 231, 236, 245, 247, 248, 250, 257–259, 261, 265, 267–269, 271, 272, 275–278, 280, 281, 283, 284, 304, 305, 309, 311, 315, 317, 319–321, 323–326, 332–342, 344, 345

laxative, 121, 122, 126, 162, 187, 188, 353

lemon, 4, 20, 30, 42, 52, 63, 67, 69, 73–78, 85, 90, 94, 97, 100, 110, 119, 125, 129, 133, 139, 140, 148, 152, 155–157, 159, 164, 165, 168, 173, 175, 176, 178–180, 184, 185, 190, 194, 199, 203, 214, 224, 228, 229, 231, 239, 244, 251, 257–259, 262–266, 268, 269, 272, 277, 279–282, 288, 294, 296, 304, 305, 309, 317, 319, 320, 322, 325, 326, 332, 334–337, 339, 341, 346

lemon verbena, 42

lemongrass, 30, 42, 52, 63, 72, 78, 90, 97, 120, 149, 157, 169, 178, 209–214, 219, 222, 229, 257, 258, 262, 265, 267, 274, 275, 282, 303, 305, 309, 313, 317, 334, 339, 342, 345

Leo, 321, 328

lesions, 64, 196, 197

lethargy, 160, 259, 278

Libra, 322, 328

lice, 64, 66, 109

limbic system, 17, 18, 256

lime, 42, 52, 140, 244

liniment, 216, 238

loneliness, 259, 279

love notes, 63

luck, 144, 153, 157, 190, 219, 286

Magellan, 182

malaria, 111

JUN - - 2017